I0413837

Food For Your Dosha

Dr. Navin Joshi & Dr. Shilpa Yerme

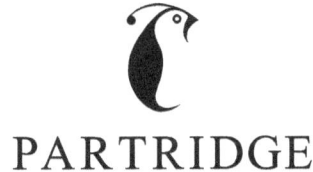

PARTRIDGE

Copyright © 2022 by Dr. Navin Joshi & Dr. Shilpa Yerme.

ISBN: Softcover   978-1-5437-0879-0
            eBook   978-1-5437-0878-3

All rights reserved. No part of this book may be used or reproduced by any means, graphic, electronic, or mechanical, including photocopying, recording, taping or by any information storage retrieval system without the written permission of the author except in the case of brief quotations embodied in critical articles and reviews.

Because of the dynamic nature of the Internet, any web addresses or links contained in this book may have changed since publication and may no longer be valid. The views expressed in this work are solely those of the author and do not necessarily reflect the views of the publisher, and the publisher hereby disclaims any responsibility for them.

Print information available on the last page.

To order additional copies of this book, contact
Partridge India
000 800 919 0634 (Call Free)
+91 000 80091 90634 (Outside India)
orders.india@partridgepublishing.com

www.partridgepublishing.com/india

Contents

Preface

We are happy to present this unique book "**Food for Your Dosha** ".

Health is the prime important thing in one's life.

In Today's world everyone is engaged with carrier, work, ambitions and many more things. We often ignore what we are eating and what is needed to our body. Prakriti a very unique concept of Ayurveda which helps in various ways to maintain health.

Diet is the first need of human.

According to Ayurved Ahar, Nidra,Bramhchrya are three pillars of human .

Food plays a crucial role in one's health as Ayurveda classics has given elaborative description on food. Acharya charka has a very special contribution in describing food. the association of food with disease, growth of children, immunity, fertility, maternal child health issues attracted attention towards the subject.

One should take food according to his body Constitution, Age, Profession, Health status, Season. if we consider all such things, it will keep equilibrium in dosha status and balance the normal physiology.

As the country is divided in many regions and states every state is having its own culture of food.

If one can take food according to his dominant dosha or prakriti it will help him to stay healthy for a long.

Food for your Dosha is knowledge feast for readers as it guides all the aspects of food. the interesting part of this book is that we have covered some unique points like properties of food, food according to age, disease wise food, body pattern wise food utensils for kitchen, colours and their impact on food and many more. Some simple easy breakfast, lunch, dinner recipes are included for readers.

We thank all who helped us for this book. Students, readers, doctors are our source of inspiration.

We thank the publication team for their kind cooperation.

We recommend this book as a reference book .

We hope this book will help out everyone and Guide what, how, when to eat.

We welcome readers suggestions.

Thanks & Regards -- Dr. Navin Joshi   Dr. Shilpa Yerme Patil

Chapter 1

Introduction

Food played a major role for human, animal and all living organism on earth.

When we look back humans have to struggle for food. during the past decades great changes have been made in the field of nutrition and disease application of it. during the earlier time man leaves by eating raw food items (fruits, vegetables, meat etc). then man noticed the food becomes tasty due to roasting it, then he started using fire for making food. in the starting he uses only roasting of meat, vegetables, afterwards he tried to make it in variety. he used water to make it easy for mastication, swallowing etc.

after second world war due to technology and media it becomes need to form associations which can look after the health issues. who, UNICEF started working to the needy people by suppling food, medical necessity? then food science started growing first they make daily requirement chart for soldiers and slowly for lay man.

as the country is divided in many regions and states every state is having its own culture of food.

the association of food with disease, growth of children, immunity, fertility, maternal child health issued payed attention towards the subject.

in ayurved food is categorised under many categories.

'food' eatable items are included in this category.

diet '– the type of food material that we consume like fruits, vegetables, milk & milk products animal products.

science of nutrition means which deals with all the aspects (physiology, chemistry, medicine) .

    diet is the first need of human.
    according to ayurved ahar, nidra,bramhchrya three pillars of human .
    ahar functions –
    food is vital power of human body.

food gives us nourishment, sweet voice, intellectual capacity, life, joy, strength all such factors depend upon food.

Chapter 2

Classification of Food

food can be classified under following categories

A. **According to Source of food**

  1. vegetable food – human body is made of variety of cell. cell requires energy, nutrition for their daily activities. the food we get from vegetable sources is known as vegetable food. (cereals, nuts, pulses etc.)
  2. animal food – milk & milk products, fish, eggs, meat can be included in this category.

B. **According to function –**

  1. body building food – proteins – proteins are required for cell development, growth, stamina, strength of cell.
  2. energy giving agents – carbohydrates – carbohydrate is required for energy of functioning of cell.
  3. protective food – fats / lipids are great reservoir of food. fats are stored in humans which can be utilised as per the requirements.

C. According to nutritional values

1. vegetables – green vegetables, fruit vegetables, are the great source of minerals and vitamins. daily intake of vegetables is required to balance nutritional status.
2. cereals – jowar, wheat, maize, oats, barley – great source of protein and carbohydrates.
3. pulses – moong dal, red gram, toor dal, chavali, rajma, massor
4. vegetables – tomatoes, potatoes, lady's finger, brinjal, beans, carrot, cucumber, cauliflower, cabbage etc.
5. fruits – banana, pomegranate, guavas, mango, grapes, oranges, apple etc
6. milk & milk products- curd, buttermilk, Paneer, cheese etc are rich source of minerals

D. **Vitamins** – vitamins are categorized as fat soluble & water soluble.

A, D E, K are fat soluble vitamins which can be stored and used . B- complex, C are water soluble vitamins daily required.

E. **Minerals** – Na, Ca, K, P,Cl all such minerals are necessary for routine metabolic activities of cells. minerals are of three types major (Ca, Mg, Na,P) minor (iron, sulphur)micro minerals (iodine, chlorine). all minerals play a vital role cellular activity like oxidation, acid-base balance, muscle-bone-teeth health.

F. According to taste (rasa)

according to ayurved tastes are of 6 types. every substances on earth is made of five elements – Prithvi, Aap, Teja, Vayu, Akash .

1. Sweet – Madhur rasa – made up of Prithvi & Jala. sweet taste is accepted universally as it is the taste of mother's milk. it is good for complexion, skin tone, hairs, full of ojas, gives strength in emaciation person, nourishes all dhatus.
   it is best used for vata, pitta person. but in excess it vitiates kapha dosha (santarpanjanya vyadhi).

it is symbol of love, sharing.

food items – rice, water, milk, wheat, honey, moong dal.

2. Sour – amla rasa – it is made up of earth & fire. it is hot & heavy stimulates vata activity. sour taste aids digestion so in India it is used for preparing food on daily basis.

   it indicates envy.

   in excess it vitiates pitta & kapha dosha.

   food items – fermented food items, yoghurt, bread, pickles, sour fruits etc.

3. Salty – lavan rasa – made up of water & fire element. it helps in salivation thereby stimulates digestion.

   it pacifies vata dosha and vitiates pitta & kapha dosha. if excess used causes greying of hair,wrinkles, baldness.

   it indicates greed.

   food items – all type of salts

4. Pungent (spicy)- katu rasa – made up of fire & air. it possesses hot, dry, light qualities. it helps in digestion. it pacifies kapha & increases pitta, vata dosha. if used excess it may cause pain, tremors thirst etc.

   it denotes passion, anger emotions.

   food items – all type spices such as clove, chilis, black pepper, ginger etc. such spices are best used in kapha disorders.

5. Bitter – Tikta rasa – it is made up of space & air. it helps in cleaning mouth, it absorbs moisture from various substances like fat, faces etc.

   if excess used it causes thirst, loss of strength etc. it pacifies kapha, pitta and vitiates vata dosha. too much use may cause fear or nervousness.

   food items – spices like turmeric, fenugreek, tea, coffee etc.

6.   Astringent- Kashaya rasa – made up of earth & air element. it constricts the oral mucosa. it vitiates vata & pacifies pitta, kapha dosha. if excess used it absorbs the moisture, constipation, blocks channels.

food items – pomegranate, tea, coffee, broccoli, cauliflower etc.

Taste – rasa	Panchmahabhut	Season – Rutu (dominance of rasa in herbs)
sweet	earth – water	Hemant
sour	earth – fire	Varsha
salty	fire – water	Sharad
pungent	fire – air	Gresham
bitter	space – air	Shishir
astringent	earth – air	Vasant

G. Panchbhautik classification –

according to ayurveda every substance or human body is made five elements. food we ingest it must be taken according to mahabhut dominance.

Panchmahabhut	attributes	functions	food items
Prithvi – earth	heavy, stable,	gives stability firmness	
Jala – water	moist, slow, heavy,	olation,	milk, water, rice, sugarcane juice
Teja – fire	dry, hot, sharp, fine, sour	digestion, transformation	chilli, long piper, spices like garlic, ginger, Asefodia
Vayu – air	dry, light, fine		
akasha – space	light, fine		

H . Trigunatmak diet – (three attributes of diet)

Satva, raja, tama these three are basic component of food. human body is made up of trigunas, every person has a different personality according to presence of three attributes . one famous quote is that "you are what you eat "the meaning is having depth. exactly what we eat it effect on our body. Sattvik food balances the mind, body, soul. pure (sattvik) food purest mind, thoughts, free from any kind of attachments. Satva is divine in nature while raja,tama imbalances mind,body, soul.

A. Sattvic food – food that is fresh, appropriate taste, which gives us energy, balances tridosha, healthy, mindful, gives physical strength. preferably this food is prepared in home with pure soul mind and full of love. Homemade food which is made by our beloved ones can be taken as sattvic food. Person who want peace, spirituality excellence in life must take this food .

Food items –

1. **Wheat** - wheat are best source of carbohydrate, can be used in variety of forms like roti, chapati, phulka, porridges.
2. **Rice** – according to ayurved old rice (basmati or rice which is grown in 60 days is good to consume. Rice is sweet in taste it nourishes tissues, can be used from 6 months of life (baby's first food is rice).
3. **Ghee –(clarified butter)**- cow's ghee is good source of satva quality. Ghee can be used daily with various food items like roti, daal, rice, porridges, laddus,halva,majority of sweet items can be made by using ghee.
4. **Milk** – milk is appreciated in ayurved classics due to its properties like sweet, nutritious, grounding rejuvenation. Milk can be used alone with spices like turmeric,cardamom, milk can be added in sweets.
5. **Moong daal (green gram)** - best among all pulses, light,tasty,balances three doshas. soup, with cooked vegetables, moong dosa, moon laddu can be used.
6. **Pomegranate** – best fruit which is good source of iron, vitamins,easy to digest. Best used in hyperacidity, ulcers,anaemia, irritable bowl syndrome, anorexia, dysentery.
7. **Banana** – sweet,tasty .nourishes all tissues, improves muscle strength. Used in debility, infertility,to gain weight.

8. **Oranges – good** for digestive problems. Best source of vitamin c. nourishes mind,soul

9. **Grapes** – sweet, cool, nourishes all tissues. Best for healing mind body. Best used in burning diseases, epistaxis, thirst, ulcers, acidity, stomach pain, gastritis.

10. **Mango – sweet**, delicious in taste, nourishes dhatu,. Best used for weight gain, low sperm count.

11. **Coconut** – sweet, nutritious, maintain fluid balance. Coconut water is best used in diarrhoea, vomiting, hypotension.

12. **Fig** – sweet, tasty, full of minerals.

13. **Dates** – sweet, nourishes all dhatu. Best to use in general debility, burning diseases, acidity, to gain weight. Rich source of iron best to use during pregnancy, postpartum periods.

14. **Peaches** – nourishes dhatus.

15. **Pears** – tasty

16. **Almond** – best source of energy, minerals, nourishes mind body, rejuvenates tissues.

17. **White sesame** – best source of iron, can be used in chutneys, laddus.

18. **Fresh cashews** – best to take with milk, rich in energy.

19. **Saffron** – give fragrance to food, pure in nature

20. **Turmeric** – best antibacterial, antimicrobial, antiviral properties. gives taste, colour to food.

21. **Coriander**- it is used as spice while making food . gives flavour to food. due to its cooling property can be used in burning diseases, ulcers, gastritis, stomach pain.

22. **Fennel** - used as a spice in Indian cooking. Flavours food, having medicinal properties. Can be used as home medicine in burning diseases, enhances digestion.

23. **Cumin** – improves taste, flavours food,used on daily basis in Indian cooking. Best carminative, digestive item.

24. **Cardamom** – it is spice with cooling property mostly used in spicy and sweet dishes also.

25. **Sweet potatoes** – sweet potatoes are mostly used during rituals or fasting period in India. Best source of energy, rich of minerals.

26. **Asparagus** – used as a vegetable .

27. **Sprouts** – according to ayurved sprouts should be consumed by cooking in less quantity.

B. Rajasic food – according to ayurved food which aggravates pitta, vata dosha is rajasic food. Rajasic food stimulates stomach fire, outward movement, aggressiveness. it is noted that when we eat such type of food our mind becomes cruel, aggressive which is one of reason of dosha aggravation.

1. **spicy** – any food which is made spicy by adding more spices, masalas, salt oil.
2. **Meat / fish** – as discussed detailed in another chapter meat aggravates raja guna in mind, mind becomes unstable so better to avoid.
3. **Pickles** – pickles are salty, oily, sour aggravate pitta, anger, violence.
4. **Tea / coffee** – tea coffee both are astringent in taste aggravates vata, pitta. several actions are noted on mind.
5. **Onion / garlic** – onions and garlics are used as spice in Indian cooking. Which are stimulant, aphrodisiac. In many parts of India people avoid to consume this as a part of custom. It is avoided during fasting, rituals.
6. **Wines** – wines are used as medicines but daily or frequent consumption in not indicated.
7. **Sour fruits** – sweet fruits are good for health but sour aggravates pitta,vata dosha. Most of citrus fruits (tamarind, guavas,
8. **Potatoes** – potatoes are used widely as rich in carbohydrates but they are rajasic according to ayurveda.
9. **Broccoli**
10. **Spinach** – it aggravates pitta dosha .
11. **Cauliflowe**r - little is good to consume but use with few spices.
12. **Sour cream / sour butter** - aggravates pitta, vata dosha and mind becomes irritable which in turn work as a Hetu (cause) for disease.
13. **Millet** – contains secondary type of qualities with few health benefits.
14. **Corn** – as it heavy dry, hard to digest, disturbs dosha.
15. **Buckwheat** –

16. **Beans** – Toor, brown lentils,

17. **kidney, black beans** -

18. **curry** – chili, spices, black pepper – aggravates raja guna and pitta dosha.

19. **Sugar / artificial sweetener / cooked honey** – all these are not recommended as aggravate pitta dosha.

20. **Brown sesame seeds** –

C. Tamasic Diet – Tama attribute is heavy & stable. The food which stale, frozen, processed, left overnight food, instant, microwave food creates confusion in mind . this further aggravates dosha.

Food items -

- Foods which make your mind dark and confused are called as tamasic food. As earlier discussed Satva Guna enlightens the Mind.
  Tamasic food is that which is cooked by using oils, instant methods. Frozen food, left overnight stale food items, meat, fish, alcohol, onions, fast food items . such type of food slows down the metabolism, lowers stomach fire and hence not good for health.

I. According to Drug

1. shaman- drugs which normalize (pacifies) the dosha ex. oil – vata,
2. kopan- drugs which vitiates dosha. yogurt – pitta vitiation
3. swasthhitkar – drugs/ food which do not interfere with dosha and can be beneficial any time. milk, moong dal, wheat balances dosha and are beneficial.

a. cereals –

1. Rice – pacifies vata, pitta, vitiates kapha dosha
2. Wheat – sweet, nourishing, healing. pacifies vata, pitta
3. Jwari Millet – Nourishing, sweet light to digest
4. Bajara – dry, hot. pacifies kapha, vata, vitiates vata dosha.
5. Satu (barley) – nutritious, helps to rejuvenate.
6. Nachani –Finger millet strengthening

7. Rajgira – Amarnath - light to digest
8. Shingada – water chest nut - good source of proteins

b. **pulses** – (lentils)

1. Toor dal – yellow pigeon peas
2. Moong dal – green gram
3. Massor dal – red lentils
4. Chana dal – spilt Bengal gram
5. Chavli – black eye beans
6. Rajma – kidney beans
7. Hari matar (vatana) – green peas
8. Urad dal – spilt skinned black gram
9. Moth – Turkish gram
10. Chori – adzuki beans

c. **vegetables** – vegetables can be divided in three categories, green vegetables, fruit vegetables, others

1. Onion – gives strength, taste. vitiates kapha, little pitta, pacifies vata
2. Potatoes- vitiates kapha, if taken excess vitiates pitta, vata also.
3. Beans – Vitiates vata (use by soaking), heavy to digest
4. lettuce -astringent use little for all three Dosha.
5. Cabbage – good for pitta and kapha. Cooked cabbage is good for vata Dosha.
6. Cauliflower-
7. Carrot – sweet, hot, vitiates pitta
8. Karela -bitter gourd – pacifies kapha, pitta, vitiates vata dosha.
9. Capsicum – simla mirch
10. Kheera- cucumber – vitiates vata, pacifies pitta
11. Chukander – beet root
12. Dhaniya- coriander
13. Tomato- pacifies vata, vitiates pitta, kapha
14. Bhindi -lady's finger- pacifies vata, pitta, vitiates kapha
15. Gavar – cluster beans –
16. Mooli- radish

17. Hara pyaz – green onion
18. Methi –fenugreek – mainly work as female health booster. pacifies
19. Palak – spinach –
20. kumbha – mushroom
21. parwal – pointed gourd
22. tohri – ridged gourd
23. Pudina – mint
24. lal mirch – red chilli
25. Kadhi patta – curry leaves
26. Ajmoda – celery
27. kaccha kela- raw banana –
28. moringa – drumstick
29. Hari Gobi, broccoli
30. Baingan – Brinjal – vitiates kapha, heavy, pacifies vata, pitta
31. Lashon- garlic- aphrodisiac, unctuous, hot, digestive, healing property, rasayan, helps in diseases like cough, fever, anorexia, piles,

d. fruits

1. Draksha – grapes
2. Amra – mango ripened mano is good for health sweet, aphrodisiac, gives strength pacifies vata, pitta dosha, vitiates kapha dosha.
3. Dadim – pomegranate – absorbent, strengthens heart, pacifies pitta
4. kela – banana
5. Chiku – sapota
6. Ananas – pineapple
7. Tarbooj – watermelon
8. Santri oranges
9. Papita -papaya –
10. Amrud – guava
11. Jambu – blackberry – absorbent, dry, pacifies kapha,pitta
12. Kathal – jackfruit
13. Seb – apple
14. Neelbadri – blueberry
15. Sarifa – custard apple- sweet,cold,pacifies pitta,re

16. khajur – dates -
17. Anjir – fig
18. Nashpati – pear
19. Mosambi – sweet lime
20. kharbuj – muskmelon- diuretic, heavy, unctuous, sweet, pacifies pitta dosha.
21. Ber – jujube – light, hot, pacifies vata,vitiates pitta,kapha
22. strawberry
23. Ganna- sugarcane
24. Shakarkand – sweet potato
25. kaitha- limonia acidissmia

Chapter 3

Concept of Prakriti

Prakriti a very basic and unique concept of Ayurved. prakriti is enumeration of body features internal as well as external. prakriti or body type can be determined by proportion of three dosha. ayurveda classified body types based on predominance of dosha. this predominance depends upon predominance of dosha is ovum and spermatozoon mean shukra and shonita. ayurveda used the term prakriti in the sense of personality. ayurveda has given stress on constitutional, temperamental, psychological and emotional aspects of personality.

Acharya charka described following factors are responsible for prakriti development.

a. Intrauterine factors – sperm, ovum, uterus
b. Extrauterine – time, season, age, seasonal regimen
   Dietic regimen, seasonal regimen, emotional conditions, fathers' behaviour are also important factor which contribute in development of prakriti.

Classification of prakriti

A. **Doshaj –**
   1. Vata
   2. Pitta
   3. Kapha
   4. Samdoshaj
   5. Vata pitta
   6. Kapha pitta
   7. Pitta vata

B. **Mansik (psychological)**
   1. Satva – 7 tyes
   2. Raja – 6 types
   3. Tama – 3 types

C. **Jatayadi –** according to race, caste, locus, age
D. **Panchbhautik –** Prithvi, aap, tej, vayu, akash

Vata prakriti characters –

Vata prakriti characters are explained according to specific attributes.

1.Ruksha (Dry) –

Alpha Sharir	– Short, Lean, Thin, body.
Apachit Sharir	– Weak, Malnourished body, emaciation.
Ruksha Sharir	– Dry Body.
Swara Dry voice	– Swara has various characters.
Pratat	– Long drawn.
Ruksha	– Dry, Hoarse voice.
Bhinna	– Broken.
Sakta	– Obstructed.
Kshama	– Low Pitch.
Jarjar	– Shaky voice, Wavy.

Mand   – Slow.

Jagruka Nidra   – Always keeping a wake (conscious) due to raja guna.

2) Laghu (Light) –

Laghu Chapal cheshta   -   Light, unsteady movements.
Laghu Chapal Ahara   -   Eats Fast.
Laghu Chapal Vihar   -   Fast action.

3) Chala (Mobile)

➤ Anavasthit Sandhi – Unstable Joints.
➤ Anavasthit bhara, Akshi, Jivha, hanu, Oshta – Unstable movements of eyes eyebrows, tongue, Jaws, Lips, Uncontrolled, Unnecessary movements of shoulders, hands and legs.

4) Bahu (abundance)

Bahu Pralapa – Over talkativeness.
Bahu kandara, Sira, Pratana – Predominant, abundance of Tendons, /veins, ligaments.

5) Sighara (Swift)

– Sighara samarambha – Quick in imitation of work (action) but doesn't complete the work.
– Sighara Kshobha – Quick irritation at the onset of morbid manifestations.
– Sighara Vikara – Symptoms are seen quickly due change in life style.
– Sighara Trasa Raga, viraga – Quick response emotions strong expressed, respond quickly for likes and dislikes.
– Sighara graham, Alpa Smruti – Quick understanding capacity quick forgetting (short memory).

6) Shita (cold)

- Shita Asahishnu – intolerance of cold things food etc.
- Pratata Shitaka – Always affected by cold things.
- Udwepaka – Shivering, cold feeling.
- Staubha – Stiffness of joints – in cold weather stiffing increases.

7) Parusha (Rough)

Parusha – Shamshru, kesha, roma, nakha – rough hairs, rough hairs of bird, other parts of body.
Parusha, Dashang Vadan, Nails, teeth, face body part become rough.

8) Vishada (non-slimy)

- Sfutita Ang Avayava – Cracked body parts, skin lips, hairs become cracked.
- Satata Sandhi shabda gamina – During movement of join production of cracking sound.

Due to all these properties of vata dosha person becomes

Alpabala	-	Weak Strength.
Alpa ayu	-	short life span.
Alpa Apathya	-	Few children.
Alpa Sadhana, dhana	-	Less accessories for living, less wealth
Adhanya	-	Unfaithful personality.

B . Pitta prakriti – characters

According to special attributes pitta characters are as below .

1) Ushna (Hot) – Ushnasaha – in tolerance of hot things. They should avoid beverages, spicy food.

Ushnamukha – Due to heat face is hot reddish coloured having pimples.
Sukumar avadata gatra – clear complex of body parts.

Prabhut piplu, vyanga, tilkalaka Pidaka – possessing Pimples, discoloration, moles, feckless on face.

Kshuta pipasavant – excessive hunger and thirst, as digestion is faster hunger and thirst is excess.

Kshipravali Parita Khalitya dosha – old age symptoms appear earlier like wrinkles, graying of hair, boldness.

Mrudu Alpa kapil kesh loma shmshru – Soft, silky, brown hairs, on body parts face beard growth slow.

2) Tikshna (Sharp)

Tikshna Prakrama – Physical Strength ability is good. Courageous personality.

Tikshna agni – Digestive power strong.

Prabhut Ashan Pana- Intake capacity for food drink's is good. Prefers liquids in diet.

Like milk, Juice, Lassi etc.

Dandshook – As digestion Capacity is good frequency of intake of food is more (glutton's habits).

3) Drava (Liquidity)

Shithil, mrudu sandhibandh mamsa – due to liquidity joint becomes loose and soft.

Prabhut Shrushta, Sweda, Mutra, Purisha – intake of food is more produce large amount of stool, urine, voiding of sweat, Urine and faces in large quantity.

Vistra (Fleshy smell) –

Putikaksha vaksha sharir gandh – Putrid rotten smell of sharir especially axilla, month, head, chest.

4) Katu Amla Rasa –

Alpashukra dhatu – As shukra is shita madhur due to Ushna, Tikshna guni Pitta less amount of shukra (semen) is produced.

Alpa Vyavaya – Sexual desire is less.

Alpa Apatya – Few childres.

Due to presence of above-mentioned qualities pitta – Prakriti Persons is –

Madhya bala – moderate strength.

Madhya Ayusha – Moderate life span.

Madhya dhyan, Vidnyan – moderate intellectual power memory grasping capacity.

Madhya vitta Upakaran – Moderate Accessories, wealth in life.

C.kapha prakriti characters

according to special attributes kapha characters are as below.

1) **Snigdha (Unctuous)** – Unctuous body parts, nails, hairs skin.
2) **Slakshna (smooth)** – Smooth body parts.
3) **Mrudu (Soft)**

Drushtisukha- pleasant look (appearance), impressive looked due to soft skin and body.

Sukumar Avadata gatra – Tenderness, clear complexion charming skin.

4) **Madhura** (sweet)– Prabhut – shukra – Abundant semen (Shukra and Kapha) are having same qualities).
   Prabhut Vyavaya – Sexual capacity is good.
   Prabhut Apatya – Greater number of children.

5) **Sara (Firm)**
   Sara Sharir – Firm body parts, compact structure of dhatu.
   Sthira Sharir – As dhatus are of good quality, body becomes compact, stable firm.
   Samhat Sharir- Compact sable body masculine structure and good immunity power.

6) **Sandra (Dense)**

Upachit Paripurna gatra – As Kaph is dense it combines body Parts. Dhatus uniformly for body become well-structured uniform.

7) **Manda (Slow)**

Manda chesnta	- Slow Action.
Manda Ahara	– Slow intake of food.
Manda Vihara	– Slow activities, movements.

8) **Stimitya (Stable)**

Asigraha Arambha – Due to stability options are sloganized. Slow imitation any work but complete the work last stage.

Asigraha, Kshobha – slow irritation.

Asigraha Vikara Respond Slow Pathogenesis of disease immunity power is good.

9) **Guru (Heavy)** – Sara Adhishit Avasthit gati-stable, no slippery gait, walks by pressing sole of feet against earth (like an elephant).

10) **Shita (colds)**

Alpa book – Due to Shita guna hunger is weak. Can control hunger easily.

Alpa Trut – Weak thirst, can control thirst.

Alpa Santap – heat related disorder are few can control anger.

Alpa Sweda – Less secretion of sweat.

11) **Vijiala (Viscos)**

Susishta sara sandhi bandhan – due to sticky, soft property kapha joints muscle tendon bones strongly, uniformly compactness in joints.

12) **Accha (Clear)**

Prassana Darshan – Happy face good looking.

Prassana Annan – Charming face looks.

Snigdh varna swara – Clear complexion, soft skin, voice.

Owing to all qualities described above kapha Prakriti persons are –

1) Balwan – Strength excellent.
2) Vasumant – Wealthy.
3) Vidyavant – Knowledgeable person.
4) Mand Vihara – Soft slow spoking actions are controlled
5) Ojasvi – Vital capacity, energy is good.
6) Shant – Peaceful Nature.
7) Ayushman – Long life Span.

Dwidoshaj prakriti characters are not specified in classics, when we examine prakriti we get an idea of the same by dominance of specific dosha characters.

Following interpretation is random ones diet depends upon stomach fire, age, work pattern, physical fitness .

Food item	Vata	Pitta	Kapha
Properties of food to prefer	Moisture, warm, nourishing, oily, heavy Sweet, sour, salty	Adequate moist, liquid, nourishing, sweet,bitter,	Dry, warm, light, pungent, bitter, astringent
Properties of food to avoid	Dry, light, pungent, bitter,astringent	Hot, spicy, salty, sour	Sweet, salty, sour, heavy, Oily, slimy
Cooking pattern preferred	Fully cooked, boiled moistened, deep fry,	Cooked, steamed, liquids	Roasting, stewing, baking, steaming
Breakfast	Heavy	Heavy	Light (can skip)
Lunch	Adequately	Heavy – (can digest)	Moderate
Evening snakes	Nutritious	Nutritious	Light (can skip)
Dinner	Adequately	Adequately	Light
Liquids in diet -	Adequately	Adequately	Less is better
Digestive power	Irregular	Regular	Low
Cereals rice	Can take adequate	Can take adequate	moderately
Wheat	Can take adequate	Can take adequate	moderately
Jowar millet	moderately	Moderately	Can take adequate
Pulses – toor	moderate	Occasional	moderate
Moong daal	Can take adequate	Can take adequate	Can take adequate
Massor	Moderate	Moderate	Moderate
Chana daal	Occasionally	Occasionally	Moderate
Urad daal	Can take adequate	Occasionally	Occasionally

Nuts – almond	Abundant	Adequate	Moderate
Cashew nut	Abundant		
Raisins	Abundant	Abundant	Moderate
Dates	Abundant	Abundant	Occasionally
Jaggery	Abundant	Moderate	Occasionally
Milk	Abundant	Moderate	Occasionally
Ghee – butter	Abundant	Abundant	Moderate
Paneer	Moderate	Occasionally	Occasionally
Buttermilk	Moderate (masala)	Moderate	Occasionally
Curd – fresh	Moderate	Occasionally	Occasionally
Green vegetables	Moderate	Occasionally	Moderate
Bakery products	Moderate	Occasionally	Occasionally
Fruits – mango	Abundant	Moderately	Occasionally
Banana	Abundant	Moderately	Occasionally
Coconut	Moderate	Abundant	Occasionally
Spices	Can use abundant	Occasional, cool spices	Moderate
Meat	Moderately	Better to avoid	Occasional
Seafood	Moderately	Better to avoid	Occasional
Water	Can use abundant – warm better	Can use abundant Cool – medicated	Moderate, warm
Sprouts	Can use occasionally (cooked)	Moderate	Moderate

As in chapter we have discussed detail plan about dosha specific diet here are summary points for all dosha.

chapter 4

Food For Your Dosha

A. Vata Dosh Prakriti –

as earlier discussed vata prakriti should plan diet for balancing vata. this can be little altered according to age, occupation, season.

key points –

1. Vata food should be quite warm, unctuous, moist, nurturing, soothing, grounding, refreshing, pleasing, heavy, satisfying.
2. Vata increases by age, autumn, cold cloudy weather, afternoon, travel time, loud noise, cold wind so avoids vata vitiating food at his time. select food accordingly.
3. As vata is irregular maintain time schedule for food. always take food in divided quantity (small meal). don't eat too much at a time. avoid mixing of food with different properties.
4. add plenty of spices, salt, oil, cook well while making food. beans must be used by soaking overnight, remove water and cook with fresh water without lid (cover). make them by using spices.
5. nuts can be used by soaking so it will become easy to digest, enhances the properties.

6. chew food well it enhances release of digestive enzymes helps in digestion.
7. avoid outside food as much as possible.
8. drink plenty of water.
9. add adequate amount of milk, oil, ghee, jaggery while making food.
10. always eat soft, warm, cooked, liquid, nourishing meal.
11. avoid stimulating drinks, cold beverages (soft drinks specially Coca-Cola) as these are carbonated which stimulates the nervous system too much. use tea coffee moderately.
12. avoid too much fasting, or irregularity in meals.
13. soups, kadhi, sar, samber can be preferred with adequate spices, salts, butter.
14. sweet sour, salty should be preferred.
15. use variety of whole grains
16. raw vegetables can be used by little steaming (add pinch of salt, jeera powder to it), it will enhance taste and easy to digest. as raw food is hard to digest and may vitiates vata dosha.
17. if wish to eat meat it must be cooked well by adding spices like ginger, garlic, cumin coriander, turmeric.
18. can take deserts adequately made up with grains, jaggery, nuts, milk, ghee creams.
19. daily 10 almonds soaked overnight skinned provide nutrition to vata people.
20. Mango, Neem, Avala haldi pickles can be used moderately. rice, urad, moong, papad can be used.
21. sea vegetables best for nourishing skin hairs,

Meal plan for vata dosha prakriti-breakfast menus –

Take regular breakfast as vata needs energy. breakfast should be nourishing, energetic. add milk, nuts (powdered, soaked preferable), juicy fresh fruits.

- Start your day with warm water, preferably you can add Nimbu, Gud, ginger in it.
- hot milk, ginger tea, soaked nuts (almonds, raisins, figs) can be taken.

Snacks-

1. whole wheat roti (bread) with plenty of butter, ghee
2. Musli, wheat flakes with warm milk, honey .
3. Sweet semolina, Upama, paratha, poha, puri(sweet, spicy, plain), idly wheat kheer,payas, dal -rice, chapati – sabji, wheat noodles, whatever fresh available.
4. It should be hot, soft, nourishing. moong, besan, wheat flour, dal laddu, halva, chikki, any available homemade snacks.

Menu Preparations

1. **Tea** – good for vata, kapha prakriti in moderate. vitiates pitta dosha.

    ingredients – 250 ml milk, 50 ml water, tea powder, sugar, jaggery as per liking, ginger piece (tea masala made up of ginger, cinnamon, clove).

    method – boil water, add tea powder, add sugar, add milk boil for a while. filter and serve.

    time required – 10 min

    persons – 2

    tea can be made by variety of procedures in india. it can be made by mixing boiled tea water and hot milk, sugar, masala etc. people use variety of masala in it as per choice. in winter masala is preferred.

2. **Ginger tea / kadha** – kadha is preferred in morning hours specially it is best in rainy, winter season for all dosha .in summer make it in mild form.

    it is best for vata, kapha. pitta should use in less quantity.

    ingredients – 200 ml water, ginger piece, sugar (honey, jaggery).

    method – boil water, add ginger, sugar, filter and serve.

3. **Mint tea** – method is same as above, instead use mint.

    best for tridosh, kapha, pitta can use frequently.

4. **Green tea** – camellia sinesis – good for tridosh, best in rainy season specially for cough, cold.
    ingredients – 200 ml water, tea leaves, honey, sugar as per likes
    method – boil water, add leaves, add honey as per liking, filter, and use.

5. **Kadha / Decoction**- kadha can be made by using variety of spices like, ginger, mint, clove, cinnamon, Tulsi, coriander, piper longum, honey, jaggery etc. this is best used in winter for all type of prakriti. it may increase pitta dosha so used mild concentration. kadha or decoction can be made by using above any ingredients. it is used from long in india as a kitchen medicine.
    kadha is used widely as a home remedy for fever, cough, cold, headache. method, quantity is same as for tea.

6. **Coffee** – coffee is astringent in taste it is better to use in moderate. it is good for kapha, vitiates pitta, vata dosha.
    ingredients – coffee powder half tsp. water 50 ml, 200 ml milk, sugar
    method – boil water, add milk, sugar, coffee, boil well, filter and use. for 1 person

7. **Poha (spicy rice flakes)**- poha is widely used for breakfast or as a snack in india.
    Poha is heavy to digest, but vata can use for a change moderately. its good for kapha, increases pitta if added spices.
    ingredients – poha (rice flakes) – 250 gm, one small chopped onion, 2 tsp. groundnuts, 4 green chilies chopped, curry leaves, 2 tsp. coriander leaves, 4 tsp. cooking oil, half tsp. cumin, mustard seeds, half tsp. turmeric, salt, half tsp. sugar. you can add potato, carrot, tomato, green peas as per choice.
    method – wash and drain poha. heat the pan add oil to it, add cumin mustard seeds to it. as it pops up add groundnuts, chili, curry leaves, onion fry it upto golden color. mix sugar salt, turmeric in poha now pour it in pan, stir well cook for 7 minutes by covering.
    decorate by coriander, coconut. you can eat it with curd, lemon juice as per liking.

8. **Upama** – (spicy semolina) it is best used for patients as its light for digestion. its good for vata, kapha, pitta can use less spicy.

   ingredients – semolina (roasted) – 250 gm, chili 4, 4 tsp oil, salt, 350 ml water, chopped onion, cumin, curry leaves, coriander, black gram dal.

   method – take oil in pan add cumin, mustard, curry leaves, chili, onion, and fry little. now add water in it let it boil, slowly with teaspoon add semolina to it as it becomes semisolid, add salt cook for 7 minutes with lid.

   decorate with coriander, coconut. you can use curd, pickle, chutney with it.

   it is adequate for 4-5 people.

9. **Sweet semolina (sheera)** – it is widely used as a prasad in India, in temples also. it is best for vata, pitta, increases kapha dosha.

   semolina – 250 gm, sugar 150 gm, water 400 ml, 5 tsp ghee, half tsp cardamom powder, 5,6 almonds, 15 raisins cashews

   method – add ghee in pan, roast semolina until it becomes golden, now add boiled water, cook for 3 minutes, now add sugar and other all ingredients. cook well for 8 minutes.

   you can add any flavor to it like pineapple, mango, banana. it is best nourishing for all dosha.

10. **Omelette** - if you are non-vegetarian or prefer eggs you must include it once a week it's a best source of protein. it's good for vata,kapha but pitta person should use little.

    ingredients – 2 eggs, 1 onion, 1 tomato, garlic, oil, salt, chill

    method – make a solution of eggs, add other chopped ingredients mix well. now add oil in pan and pour the solution in it, cook for 3 minutes, omelet is ready to serve. you can eat with chapati.

11. **Thalipeeth** – multigrain – flat bread – nourishing for vata dosha. pitta, kapha may use moderately.

    thalipeeth is a favorite dish of Maharashtra. it can be made by multigrain like wheat, jowar, bajara, besan, moong. you can prepare (bhajni) by taking all grains in equal quantity, roast them and grind, now this can be used anytime for thalipeeth .

ingredients – any available grain flour 100 gm, onion, cumin powder, coriander, garlic, ajwain (carom seed) powder, chili powder, salt, oil

method – take flour, add all the ingredients, add hot water as required to make Dough. now make it in round shape with the help of roti roller by applying oil cook well in pan by covering lid. add oil as per choice. now it is ready to eat. It is widely used as a tiffin menu for school, easy to make, tasty dish.

12. **Dhirdi** – rice flour crepes – it is famous dish made in kokan, malvan, Marathwada region of India. easy and nutritious for dosha.
    ingredients – rice flour- 100 gm, water, salt, oil,
    method- take rice water add adequate water to make it semisolid solution, add salt mix well. apply oil to pan and pour solution in it cook for 4 minutes, ghavan is ready to eat, can be eaten with green chutney, sauce, curd as per liking.

13. **laddu** – laddu is a festive dish in India, very nutritious best for vata, pitta prakriti. as it is sweet vitiates kapha dosha.
    ingredients – besan (gram flour), sugar powder, ghee, cardamom, nuts
    method – take besan flour in pan roast well on low flame (orange color) by adding ghee in it. now cool and add sugar powder, nuts as per choice mix well and make it in round shape. it can be used as morning, evening snack. best used during travelling.
    laddu can be made by wheat flour, moong flour, nachani, barley, semolina, Maida, Khobar etc. with same procedure.

14. **groundnut chikki** (nose berry, mud apples) - – chikki is nourishing Indian sweet dish good for vata, pitta. little used in kapha prakriti.
    ingredients – roasted groundnuts 200 gm, jaggery 200 gm, ghee- 2 tsp.
    method – make syrup of jaggery by heating, add nuts in it and transfer it in plate roll it evenly, after cooling cut into cubes (slabs).

chikki can be made by, cashews, coconut, nuts, rice flakes, puffed rice, sesame, almond, pistachio with same procedure.

lunch menus for vata person –

1. **Rotis-** Bread – Roti is the main course food in India. it can be made by wheat flour, jowar, bajara. all these are good for vata, pitta dosha. bajari vitiates pitta dosha, best for kapah & vata. vata, pitta should always use fresh warm roti with ghee, butter. kapha should avoid oil ghee with roti, fulkas are best for kapha.

   a. wheat roti –

       ingredients – 200 gm – wheat flour, salt, water
       take flour in a dish add salt, little oil, adequate water to make soft Dough. make small bolls and with the help of roti roller make round or triangle rotis, roast in pan with ghee or oil.

   b. jowar roti – same procedure but oil is not used for it. it is mostly used in Maharashtra, kokan, Karnataka.

   c. bajara roti – same procedure mostly used in winter season, in Gujrat used on daily basis. sesame, salt, ghee is applied to make it nutritious. vata can use with ghee, pitta use in little, kapha can use without ghee.

2. **parathas** – parathas are made up of vegetables like spinach, potato, cabbage, Methi, Mooli, carrot etc. parathas can be used as a breakfast menu or lunch menu. in Himachal Pradesh aloo paratha is eaten with yogurt, butter.

   a. Potato Paratha – it is good for vata, pitta, kapha may use in moderate quantity.

       ingredients – boiled potatoes 5, wheat flour- 250 gm, oil, chili, salt, cumin powder, coriander, turmeric, lemon juice 10 drops.

method – peel of potatoes and make soft paste add salt, chili, lemon juice, turmeric, cumin's. make soft dove of flour. now take small boll of flour add Smashed Potato and cover it well now roll and make roti. roast well by applying ghee for 4 minutes. paratha can be eaten with yogurt, butter, pickle, chutney, sauces.

b. Spinach Paratha – same procedure is followed as given above. good for vata, pitta for kapha without ghee good.

c. Cabbage Paratha – good for vata, pitta,

d. Green Gram Paratha- good for vata, pitta kapha without ghee.

e. Sweet Paratha / Dashmi – sweet paratha is widely used as a travelling menu. it is healthy in winter season. best for vata, pitta, little used in kapha dosha.

ingredients – wheat flour 200 gm, water, sugar powder or jaggery 100 gm, ghee, salt, cardamom
Method – if jaggery is using make a syrup of it, add flour in it to make dove. make rotis and roast with ghee.
for sugar – mix with flour add ghee and make a dove. make small rotis and roast with ghee.
by using jaggery we can get iron & minerals.

3. **Puri** - puris are used moderately in Indian kitchen specially for festive purposes. puris are made of wheat flour mainly. vata can use frequently but kapha, pitta use in less quantity.

a. plain puri –

ingredients – 250 gm wheat flour, salt, oil for frying
method – make Dough with water, add salt. make small bolls, with the help of roti roller make small round puris, fry on high flame. use it with cooked vegetables, pickles, chutneys, curries.

b. masala puri – same procedure but we can add soft cooked vegetables like, spinach, methi, tomato, spices like cumin, sesame, chill, coriander etc. it increases pitta, good for kapha, vata.

c. sweet puri - it can be made by using jaggery, red gourd, carrot with same procedure.

4. **vegetables** – vegetables are best used along with roti in India. they are the rich source of vitamins & minerals. vegetables can be made by frying, gravy type using masalas. in every region it is used by different methods.

   a. lady's finger - this vegetable is widely used in Indian kitchen. good for all doshas. if we use more spices, it may increase pitta dosha.

   ingredients – 250 gm lady's finger (washed & dried), one onion, 1 tsp. chili powder, pinch of turmeric, salt, mustard seeds, cumin, coriander, lemon juice 5 drops, curry leaves method – cut vegetables as per your choice (round, long). heat pan add oil, add one by one mustard, cumin, onion turmeric fry well, add chili, salt, any masala, vegetables cook well. now add pinch of sugar, lemon juice, decorate with coriander.

   b. baingan (brinjal) masala – usually procedure is same for all, you can add any type of masala (coconut powder, groundnut powder, gram flour) as per your choice. garlic, ginger paste, dhania powder, fenugreek can be used for change. good for vata, kapha, but pitta may use little spices.

   c. baingan bharta – special dish of winter specially used in Maharashtra. in this roasted baingan are garnished with masala and cooked, served with bajara roti.

   d. cabbage vegetable- we can make it simply by cooking, red chili, green chilis can be used as per choice. we can add masoor dal, green peas, tomatoes for change. good for kapha, pitta it increases vata dosha.

e. cauliflower vegetable- same method as per cabbage. it's good for all doshas.

f. potato vegetable- potato vegetable can be made with red or green chili, green peas, tomatoes, black masala. potato green vegetable is best used with chapati, puri, dosa, uttapa.

g. capsicum vegetable – it is prepared same by above method.

h. gavar - cluster beans – prepared same as above mentioned.

i. tomato vegetable- it is best used with chapati, puri. it can be made by adding onions as per choice.

j. spinach vegetable- for leafy vegetables we must wash neatly.

ingredients – spinach 250 gm, onion, moong dal, oil, salt, chili, turmeric, mustard seed, cumin
method – cut vegetable in small pieces. heat the pan add oil, add mustard, cumin let it pop up, add onion, salt, chili, add moong dal cook for 5 minutes. add chopped spinach cook for 4 minutes.
you can use masoor, chana, toor dal for preparing vegetable. it is best for all doshas. panner or butter added as per choice. besan can be used to make this vegetable.

k. fenugreek vegetable – prepared same as mentioned above. it increases pitta, good for vata and kapha. best used in women in post-natal stage.

l. Mustard leaves vegetable – Sarso ka saag is favorite dish used in Panjab, Himachal Pradesh in winter. it increases pitta dosha best for vata, kapha dosha.

m. Green Onion – it is prepared same as above.

n. Gravy Vegetables – vata can use gravy vegetables as it requires spices in diet. pitta should avoid it as it is processed with masala. kapha can use moderately.

gravy preparation – ingredients – Onions, Garlic, Ginger, Coriander, Cumin, Dhania, cinnamon, Marich, saffron, Dalchini, Coconut, cloves, black pepper. roast chopped onion, add other all the ingredients except coriander to it. roast well. then make a paste with mixer. this masala is used for any gravy vegetable like baingan, potato, tomato, paneer, chole, green peas, sprouted beans.

5. **Curries / Daal** – Daals or curries are best eaten with rice or roti.

usually Toor dal, moong dal, urad dal are used daily. as all pulses are good source of protein good for vata. little used in pitta, kapha. moong daal is best for all doshas.

daal is prepared by using tomatoes, mango powder, kokum, tamarind, jaggery for taste. we can use sambar masala, or any other spices as per choice. daal should be prepared by cooking well with pan or pressure cooker.

a. Toor daal – yellow pigeon peas – it is widely used in India. it is best eaten with south Indian dishes like idly, Dosa, uttapa. good for vata, kapha, increases pitta dosha.

ingredients – 150 gm daal, one onion, curry leaves, salt, chili, oil mustard, cumin, coriander, asafetida (if likes), jaggery, method – cook daal in cooker. heat the pan add oil, add curry leaves, mustard, cumin, onion fry well adds chili, asafetida, salt, and cooked daal mix well cook for 5 minutes. you can add tomato, tamarind as per liking.

b.   moong daal – it can be prepared with same process. moong daal is best for all doshas. it can be cooked by using green chilis.

c.   Masoor daal – it is used occasionally. prepared same as indicated above. it is good for vata, kapha, increases pitta.

d.   Urad daal – black gram daal - it is prepared same, but black masala can be used. it is especially good in winter season as it is heavy to digest. best for kapha dosha, moderately used in vata dosha, increases pitta dosha.

Sprouts – according to ayurveda sprouts (usal, beans) must used in less quantity as hard to digest. for vata it can be prepared by using spices and used in small quantity. moong sprouts are good for all dosha. green peas (vatana) increase vata dosha, causes constipation.

Rice – rice is widely used in India. it is used from early stage of life, it is the first food of childhood. rice are available in variety, basmati, indrayani, Kolam, chinur, kesar are some varieties.

according to ayurved shashtisali rice is good for health, unpolished rice is good for health. acharya charka explained mahashali (basmati) is good for health, but old rice is much more beneficial for strength (old for 6- 8 months), new rice increases kapha, pitta develops Aam dosha. Rice can be used any time it is sweet, sattvic diet it is recommended for everyone. but as increases kapha dosha little used in kapha or can be used by roasting.

rice water is best used for stimulating Agni (appetizer) in diseased person. Rice is easy to digest.

Rice is eaten with daal, curries, samber, curd, milk roti.

Rice can be prepared in variety, plain rice, curd rice, ghee rice, jeera rice, Pulao, biryanis', spinach rice, tomato rice, khichari, green peas rice.

a. steam rice – best for vata dosha. Sweet, nourishing, dhatuvardhak.

Ayurved advised to cook rice in pan with lid & off lid . but now a days most of the time pressure cooker (steamer) is used to save time.

b. Jeera rice – jeera rice is good for pitta & kapha, little used in vata prakriti.

Ingredients – boiled / cooked rice - 200 gm, jeera 2 tsp., oil, ghee, salt, coriander, green chili
Method – cook rice well, heat the pan add oil or ghee as per choice. Add jeera, curry leaves, add cooked rice salt, mix well cook for 3 minutes. Decorated with coriander.

c. Pulao / vegetable rice – it is best for tridoshas. We can add vegetables according to choice.

Ingredients – 200 gm basmati rice, water, salt, oil, curry leaves, coriander, turmeric, cinnamon, carrot, peas, potato, tomato, capsicum, cloves, cashews, onion
Method – boil the rice in pan. heat the pan, add oil, add all the ingredients one by one mix well cook for 3 minutes, add rice mix well cook for 5 minutes. We can use cooked vegetables directly. Decorate with cashews, coriander. we can serve it with raita, curd, daal.

d. Curd rice – curd rice is special dish in south India. Best for vata dosha, may increase pitta, kapha.

As it prepared with same process. take steam rice, heat pan, add oil, cumin, add rice salt, off the gas, now add curd as per choice. As curd is not heated, we have to off the gas. Use Fresh curd.

e. Tomato rice – it is good for vata kapha, increases pitta. it is made by adding chopped tomatoes, salt, onion, ghee, oil .

f. Spinach rice – it is another variety of rice, tasty,nutritious, dish. Take fresh spinach, wash and cook for 3 minutes make paste. Now by heating oil in pan add paste of spinach other ingredients as per choice, cook for 5 minutes. Garnish by coriander.

g. Green peas rice – this is best for kaph, pitta, increases vata dosha. It is best used in winter season. process is same use peas in adequate quantity.

h. Khichari – salty porridge khichari is a staple food in India, widely used as evening meal. good for vata, pitta increases kapha dosh.

Method 1-

Ingredients – variety of pulses, vegetables can be used as per choices.
200 gm rice, onion, garlic, curry leaves, coriander, coconut, cumin, mustard, oil, salt, chili, 50 gm moong beans,
Method – heat the pan add oil, other ingredients slowly,stir well add water, boil it well add salt, chili, add rice cover the lid, cook on low fire for 7 minutes. Decorated with coriander, coconut, serve hot. It can be best eaten with ghee
Method – 2 khichari made up of moong daal is best food used widely in Agni Mandya, fever,cough, cold,children's, old age persons. This simple khichari is best food as wholesome diet in every condition. It is best for tridosha.
Ingredients – moong daal 100 gm, rice – 100 gm, water, salt, cumin, ghee, oil
Method – heat the pan – add little amount of ghee or oil, add cumin, add water salt boil then pour rice in it, cover the lid, cook well for 7-8 minutes on low flame. You can made this as per your choice, for old persons, children in liquid form easy

to digest, it is best when eaten with ghee, which stimulates stomach fire.

Instead, moong, Toor daal, masoor daal can be used.

6. **Salads** – salads are not much more suits vata prakriti, but as it is having nutritional value one must include in diet. Salads can be best eaten by little steaming, sprinkle salt, cumin powder to it so it becomes easy to digest.

For making salads if likes little oil is used as a tadka. Chop the vegetables, add salt, sugar, groundnut powder, coriander in it, mix well and preferred with afternoon meals.

a. Cucumber – as it is cooling it increases vata dosha. if we use fresh and by steaming its good for all dosha. usually, people keep all the vegetables in freeze but its not good for health. Cucumber is good for pitta dosha, increase kapha if excess used.

b. Tomato – tomatoes are widely used in kitchen. As they are sour and sweet little is good for vata, pitta increase, good for kapha.

c. Cabbage – cabbage is good for tridosha.

d. Carrot – good for all dosha

e. Onions – raw onions are widely used as a salad, best used during summer season. Onions are good for vata, kapaha, increase pitta. but as they are tamasic it should be avoided during rituals, or practicing yoga.

f. Spring onion salad – it best cooling dish in summer season.

g. Beet salad – good for tridosha.

7. **Raita – koshimbir/ kachumber** – in India kachumber is widely preferred due to its benefits. It is made by using tomatoes, cucumber, carrot onion . It can be eaten with bread, roti. it good source to maintain water level and for nourishing dhatus. For making raita fresh curd is utilized. curd is good probiotic so it helps in digestion.

   a.   Cucumber raita – it increases kapha, good for vata, pitta.

   Ingredients -
   200 gm cucumber, curd – 40 gms, salt, sugar,10 gm coriander, dhania powder
   Method – washed cucumber you can use by grating or by cutting in small pieces as per choice. After grating it should be used immediately as it becomes moistened. add all other ingredients, you can give tapering with cumin & mustard. You can add chopped onion to this also.

   b.   Mix raita – for making mix kachumber you can use onion, tomato's, carrot, pomegranate seeds, cabbage as per choice.

   c.   Carrot raita – it is best for vata, pitta increase kapha dosha. same method used as mentioned above.

   d.   Cabbage raita – it is good for tridosha. We can use cabbage by little cooking as it is hard for chewing.

   e.   Pineapple raita – it increases vata, kapha, good for pitta.

8. **Pickles –** Vata prakriti persons can use adequate pickles in diet. In India making pickles in summer season is like ritual. Indian women are fond of making it in variety. In every state it is made by different methods. Most of pickles increase pitta, moderately good for kapha .pickles can be used with roti, bread, thalipeeth, Dosa. For preserving pickles vinegar is used so it becomes pitta genic.

a. Mango pickle – it liked very much by Indian people.

Ingredients – unripe mangoes ½ kg, turmeric, red chili – 50 gm, salt, mustard seeds (powder) – 2 tsp, fenugreek seeds 1 tsp. oil 150 ml

Method- after washing cut mangoes as per your choice in small pieces. Heat oil in pan – add mustard, turmeric, fenugreek seeds, off the gas . after cooling add chili, salt in it (in some parts of India chili, salt, turmeric, all spices are mixed with mango pieces). Mix well and keep in tight container preferably made of chini - Mitti (porcelain) or glass.

b. Lemon pickle – same process should by followed. It is good for vata Dosha, increases kapha, pitta.

c. Ginger pickle – it best for tridosha, if excess used pitta increases. For vata it is best to use regular. Same process should be followed.

d. Amla – pickle – it is best for all doshas. Amla pieces are used for making pickle. it is best rejuvenating for vata prakriti.

e. Sweet mango pickle – sweet pickle is best for vata, pitta prakriti. It is made by adding sugar or jaggery with same process. It can be made fresh in mango season as a best cooling menu for summer season

f. Sweet lemon pickle – it is best for vata prakriti, increase pitta, kapha.

g. Mix vegetable pickle – it is best for vata prakriti. Increases kapha, pitta. this can be prepared fresh, we can add carrots, cucumber, gavar, ginger with same masalas we can prepare this.

9. **Chutney** - chutneys are used widely as an alternative for vegetables in India or as a side menu. Chutneys are good for vata, kapha

as having spices. Increases pitta dosha. Dry & wet chutneys are preferred as per the need. dry chutneys are served along with meals. In Maharashtra groundnut chutney is mostly preferred and can be eaten with roti, bread, puri. Wet chutneys are also used with puri, roti, bread, Dosa, idly, parathas, rice.

i.   Dry chutneys-

a.   Groundnut chutney – it is good source for protein best for vata, kapha. Pitta use little. Dry chutneys are best made by using khalva (mortal)

Ingredients – 100 gm roasted groundnuts, garlic 10 cloves, red chili, cumin, salt.
Pound or grind all ingredients well and use. preferably use within 15 days .
b. sesame seed chutney- good for vata, kapha., increases pitta. 50 gm sesame seed it is made same as above mentioned.

b.   Coconut chutney – it is best for vata, kapha, increases pitta dosha. grate dry coconut or we can use fresh coconut also. Prepare with same process. Fresh coconut chutney should be used for a day only. Dry coconut for 10 days .

c.   Linseed / flax seed chutney – atasi in ayurved is balya, estrogenic. It balances vata dosha, increase pitta, kapha. Prepare with same method.

d.   Karal / Niger seed – it is widely used in Maharashtra, Karnataka, Andhra Pradesh.

It is having different taste. Good for vata dosha.

a.   Mix daal chutney – it can be made with daals like red gram, red lentil daal, black gram daal, moong daal by same process. It is specially made during marriages in Maharashtra, Karnataka.

It is known as metkut, used with rice, roti. In south India it is used with idly, Vada, rice.

ii. wet chutneys – wet chutneys are used widely for chat like pani-puri, bhel, sandwiches.

a. Mango chutney – it is best for vata, kapha prakriti, increases pitta dosha. Mango chutney best used with roti, parathas, rice.

Method 1 - Ingredients – 50 gm raw mangoes, 100 gm onion, 25 gm groundnuts, red chili, salt, cumin, jaggery 1 tsp.
Mix all the ingredients with the help mortal or mixer grind well . you can give tadka with oil if preferred or can use as raw. Best eaten with jowar roti, chapati.
Mango chutney method 2- ingredients – raw mangoes, salt, jaggery cumin seed powder. Best for vata, kapha, increases pitta dosha.
Make small pieces of mangoes. heat the pan and boil mangoes, add jaggery, salt, cumin powder cook for 5 minutes. it becomes semisolid due to cooking. best used with roti, parathas, sandwiches. You can make without cooking by grinding all the ingredients.
Method 3 – you can make this by grating mangoes add salt, red chili, and mix well. best for vata, kapha increase pitta dosha.

b. Khajur chutney – best for vata, pitta, increases kapha dosha. It can be eaten with roti, parathas, puri, sandwiches.

Ingredients – 200 gm khajur, red chili, salt, dhania powder

Method – remove the seed of khajur or use seedless. Cook khajur and make a paste, now add salt, chili in it and make thickness as per choice by adding hot water. you can add tamarind for taste in it which can be used for chat (bhel, pani-puri).

c.   Tamarind chutney – best for vata, kapha, increases pitta dosha.

Ingredients – 200 gm tamarind other ingredients same as above. cook tamarind, add salt, chili, dhania powder mix well use as per your choice with roti, for sandwiches. You add jaggery, khajur to reduce sourness of it.

d.   Mint chutney – it is good for vata, kapha increases pitta dosha.

Ingredients – 50 gm mint leaves, coriander 40 gm, salt, red chili (green chili may used),mustard seeds, turmeric, sugar, oil 2 tsp
Method - Mix all the ingredients well by mixer, give tadka with oil . can be used with parathas, sandwiches, chapati, bread, dhokla, chats.

e.   Coriander chutney - best for all three doshas.

Ingredients – chopped coriander 100 gm, green chili -4 pieces, salt, curry leaves, mustard, turmeric, cumin, sugar
Method – mix all and grind with mixer, heat the pan, add oil, add mustard, cumin let it pop up, add this oil in mixture, mix well and serve.

f.   Garlic chutney – it is best for vata, kapha prakriti, increases pitta dosha.

Ingredients – garlic cloves 50 gm, salt, cumin, red chili.
Method – mix well and grind in mixture, chutney is ready.

10. **Papad** – classical reference of papad is given in bhavprakash kritaann varg . papad is used as good appetizer, carminative, digestive agent. In India variety of papads are made specially in summer season. All type of pulses like black gram daal, red gram daal, moong daal is used along with spices. Usually, daily intake is not recommended as it develops acidity in body.

a. Urad papad – black gram papad – mash is heavy to digest, good for vata, kapha increases pitta dosha.

Ingredients – 200 gm urad daal powder, salt, asafoetida, baking soda (sarjika kshar),water
Method – make fine powder of daal . mix all ingredients with water make a dove. Keep for 1 hour, again mix well now make small bolls. With the help of roti roller roll the boll evenly in round shape. Plastic sheets can be used. After making dry well in shed – for 2,3 days (direct drying in sunshine is avoided as the shape becomes irregular). after complete drying store in a container. It can be used for 1-2 yrs.
Roasted papads are good instead of frying. We can use papads by garnishing with masala like chopped onions, tomatoes, coriander, salt, chili. best used with meal as appetizer or evening snack.

b. Moong daal papad – best for all doshas. same process is applied for moong papad.

c. Mix papad – papads are made with equal amount of moong & urad daal. Other process is same.

11. **Other beverages with lunch**

a. Butter milk – mattha – in ayurved takra is prime drink which is very useful to our body. It is best for vata, little used in kapha, pitta prakriti. Use always fresh, in Indian culture it is used on daily basis. As per choice we can make it with spices also.

Ingredients – fresh curd 100 gm, salt, cumin powder, coriander ginger garlic paste, adequate water
Method – buttermilk is prepared by churning curd with water as per liking. Add all the ingredients as per choice. Generally, it is used by adding salt & cumin powder for taste, it becomes easy to digest.

b. Masala buttermilk / mattha – it is spicy buttermilk you can add spices like dhania, cumin, black piper powder in it. It is best for vata, kapha, increases pitta dosha.

c. Sweet buttermilk / lassi – take buttermilk as per your requirements add sugar, little salt, churn with churning rod. best if used little cool. A preferred drink in summer which is made in flavours by adding pulp of mango, pineapple or kesar.

d. Curd – some people use curd along with lunch, it is good for vata but should consume fresh one. Curd is not much good for pitta, kapha. According to ayurved curd is avoided during nights.

In India curd is preferred to consume with rice, chapati, roti, puri or parathas. Best to use by adding little salt or sugar. Curd sugar is included as a ritual for a good start. Curd sugar is eaten as sweet dish .in south India curd rice is famous dish.

12. **Sweets in meals** – vata can use sweets regularly as they are dhatu nourishing. But use moderately to maintain health.

a. Semolina – sheera – it is best dish for pacifying vata, it can be used any time in a day. Process is given above. With same process wheat flour sheera can be made good for vata,pitta but increases kapha dosha.

b. Kheer – payas – porridges – in ayurved Samhitas payas are described for medicinal purposes also, it is made of various varieties. It is best used for children's, old age persons, lactating women, for patients. In garbhini paricharya (pregnancy care)

1. vermicelli payas – vermicelli's are made of wheat flour in India it is made in summer season and can be stored for a year.

50 gm vermicelli, sugar or jaggery 30 gm. ghee, raisins, cardamom powder ½ tsp., milk 300 ml

Process – roast the vermicelli by adding ghee on low flame now add milk, sugar cook add other ingredients cook for 2 minutes serve hot. Saffron, cashews almonds can be added as per choice.

2.   Rice payas – same process is followed. Good for vata, pitta, increases kapha. roast the rice make powder cook by adding milk, sugar. rest you can add nuts for taste.

3.   Semolina payas – best for vata, pitta. Process is same roast with ghee and boil with milk add sugar, nuts as per choice.

4.   Wheat payas – it is famous dish in Maharashtra, Karnataka as huggi. it is made by special variety of wheat (jod gahu), but can be made by any type of wheat.

Ingredients – crushed wheat – 100 gm, ghee, milk 400 ml, sugar or jaggery coconut, cardamom powder
Process - little roast wheat with ghee, cook the wheat in water add milk sugar, jaggery, coconut make it semisolid . it can be eaten with chapati, puri. Some people use by adding milk, ghee in it.

5.   Louki kheer – Bottle gourd – it is healthy and delicious dish for all but kapha may take rarely. Take louki and grate it, roast and cook in milk, add, sugar, flavours in it.

6.   Carrot halva- it is good for vata, pitta, increases kapha. Best dish of winter.

Ingredients – 500 gm carrot, sugar 200 gm, milk 250 ml, khoya 100 gm, cardamom, cashews, almonds, ghee
Method – grate the carrots, roast little on ghee add, sugar, and cook well for 20 minutes add other ingredients, you can add raisins, saffron as per your choice. Serve hot, it can be used for 2-3 days.

1. Basundi – in moderate quantity good for vata, pitta increases kapha. Excess is not good for tridosha, hard to digest sometimes it may cause loose motions.

    Ingredients – 2 litre milk, 700 gm sugar, nuts, cardamom
    Method – boil milk on low flame till it turns into thick. Add sugar, nuts, boil again as per your choice of thickness. Serve hot.

2. Moong Daal halva – best dish for all doshas. nourishing to all dhatus.

    Ingredients – Moong Daal 500 gm, sugar 250 gm, khoya 100 gm, milk 100 ml, 500 gm ghee, nuts, saffron
    Method – Take moong and soak it in water at least for 4 hours, drain, grind with mixer. Heat the pan and paste, add ghee roast on low flame till turns into pink colour, add milk, sugar cook for 3 minutes, garnish with nuts. It can be used for 7 days.

3. Sweet roti – Dashmi – it is famous during journey as they are soft and tasty.

    Ingredients – wheat flour 200 gm, sugar or jaggery -100 gm, salt, cardamom, ghee,milk – 80 ml
    Method - take milk add sugar or jaggery mix well, add adequate flour to make dove add salt, cardamom,ghee make a soft dove. Make bolls and roll by using roti roller roast with ghee.

    Evening snacks – During evening time vata people can take tea, milk, seasonal fruits, or any beverages as per choice. Growing children's or many people need evening snacks. according to ayurved evening meal should be taken earlier upto 7 pm. So if needed one can take evening snacks as per your stomach fire.

    For vata we should always prefer nourishing diet. Any morning breakfast dish, like laddu, chapati with curry, puri, chivada, poha can be used for snacking. Some different menus are suggested for vata

a.i. Chivda – 1 - it is best used as a appetizer. in India it is preferred as evening snacks.

Ingredients – puffed rice – 250 gm, oil, red chili, salt, turmeric, curry leaves, mustard, cumin, dhania powder, lemon juice, sugar Method – heat the pan add oil, add mustard, cumin seeds let it pop up, turn off gas add other ingredients mix well now, add puffed rice mix well on low flame. It is spicy can be used with chopped onion, tomatoes, coriander as a dry bhel. Best nourishing snack but pitta kapha may use little.

ii. chivada – 2 – it is made of poha (pruthuka) rice flakes. According to ayurved literature it is heavy hard to digest so one can consume little as may cause constipation. It increases kapha dosha, if spicy increase pitta also.

Process is same as above.

Iii . Jowar lahi – it is preferred for vata, kapha. It contains calcium minerals. Made with same process.

b. fruits – any seasonal fruit vata can prefer specially figs, dates, mangoes, chickoo, oranges, grapes, papaya preferably used.

d. beverages – tea, coffee in little quantity grain biscuits can be used. buttermilk with salt, lassi, any fruit juice, sugarcane juice can be taken.

e. nuts – soaked almonds, figs, raisins can be used

,or in powder form with milk can be consumed.

f. khajur (Date) shake best used as it gives nourishment. banana smoothies, apple smoothies, sweet potatoes, coconut water are best used.

g. popcorn, homemade Shankar Pala, chakli, shev, pea nut chikki, chapati roll (Franky made up with vegetables).

h. pakora – bhaji – as it is fried food not much recommended but can be used rarely. It is famous in India as a evening snack. It can be made with any vegetable like potato, brinjal, cauliflower, green chili, spinach, Methi, coriander, Paneer, cheese.

method 1 – chick pea flour – 200 gm, onion chopped, salt, red chili, baking soda, turmeric, coriander, water, oil. take flour in bowl add, add salt, chili, turmeric, soda (instead soda you can add hot oil 2 tsp) mix well add water to make batter. Add onion pieces, coriander and put in heated oil, fry well (upto become orange red crispy) . drain and put on paper use hot with sauce, mint chutney.

method 2- pakoras can be made with any other vegetables with same recipe. Spinach, potato, panner, cheese good for vata dosha.

Evening Meal – it is best to take dinner earlier upto 7 pm.

light meal is good for vata dosha.

In evening time chapati, cooked vegetable, soup, rice is preferred. the diet should be simple. Due to working pattern most of the family make brunch meal in afternoon and full meals in evening. but it is hard to digest heavy meal in evening. Rice, chapati, vegetables recipes already given.

Vata must prefer milk in evening, it is good for strength as well helps for sound sleep. As vata sleep is irregular so vata should include some nourishing before going to bed.

A. **Soups** – soups can be preferred even in afternoon lunch but best in evening time. Soups are best appetizer for every person, for vata hot soup is really a good choice. Soups are preferred for patients, old persons as a best nourishing drink.

I. tomato soup – good for vata peoples. Kapha, pitta person uses little.

250 gm - red tomatoes, I big onion, salt, cumin powder, black pepper powder, sugar, ghee, or butter

Method – wash tomatoes, cut and boil, heat the pan add ghee, onion, salt, sugar boiled tomatoes cook for 5 minutes. Now blend the mixture. you can add hot water as per your choice to make thin. Add butter or ghee or cream if likes serve hot.

1. spinach soup – it is good for vata, pitta without ghee for kapha dosha. Same process should be followed to make spinach soup.
2. Mix vegetable soup – it is good for all doshas. you can use carrots, French beans, green peas, tomatoes, capsicum as per choice. wash boil, add spices, ghee blend and use.
3. Moong daal soup – it is best for all doshas, as wholesome drink for low stomach fire. best used in any condition.

    Ingredients – 100 gm moong daal (with chilka may be used), salt, red chili, ghee, black pepper powder.

    Method – boil daal in water till it turns soft, add turmeric. heat the pan add ghee, add salt, cumin seeds, mix daal, pepper powder add adequate hot water to make thin cook well & serve.

4. Toor daal soup – good for vata, kapha, increases pitta. It is made as above method of moong daal soup
5. Black gram soup – it is heavy to digest best for vata, increases pitta, kapha should use less. It nourishes dhatus.
6. Kadhi – buttermilk soup – it is famous dish in Maharashtra, Gujrat, Rajasthan. kadhi is used with rice, khichari, chapati. It is best for vata, pitta, aggravates kapha dosha.

    Ingredients – buttermilk 200 ml, besan 50 gm, salt, red chili, cumin, oil, coriander, curry leaves, asafoetida

Method – add besan an in buttermilk and make thin as you like. Heat the pan add oil, cumin, asafoetida let it pop up, add curry leaves, add buttermilk OR ghrita, salt, chili let it boil for 5 minutes. Serve hot by adding coriander.

You can make without adding turmeric. Some people make it without heating as in ayurved heating buttermilk is not advised. For that use boiled water make batter of all spices along with buttermilk add besan mix well. Now make tadka and pour into batter mix well and use.

7. Saar – Saar is thin syrup of vegetables likewise soup. Saar are good for vata, kapha people.

    a. Tomato Saar – take 200 gm tomatoes cook well smash. Put the pan on gas add adequate oil afterword's add Hing, cumin, mustard seeds, coriander, curry leaves, tomato paste . after little roasting add adequate water to make thin saar . Add salt, sugar, chili, cook well and serve hot. it can be eaten with rice, khichari.

    b. Tamarind Saar – it is best for vata, little for kapha, increases pitta.

    Make with same process remove seeds of tamarind and add some jaggery to increase flavour.

B . Pitta Dosh Prakriti –

As pitta is hot, sharp stomach fir is good, digestive capacity of pitta is good. Pitta's hunger should be satiated regularly. if not satisfied regularly it may turn into irritation. anger.

key factors – pitta should use, cool, dry, light property food.

General rules for pitta –

1. strictly avoid fasting
2. use cool food, even avoid tea, coffee any hot potency food material.
3. pitta should avoid pungent, sour, salty food, sweet, bitter, astringent is good for pitta.
4. dont eat when angry or irritated, eat with calm mind.
5. avoid spicy food but can use in moderately in winter season.
6. pitta person prefer vegetarian diet, as non veg diet is heavy, hot pitta may avoid or if wish to eat take preferably in cold season in low quantity.
7. pitta shouldn't eat bakery items, packed food, salty, instant hybrid grains.
8. pitta is having a glutton's habit, as they can digest, they can eat but take food which is neutralizing pitta.

Cooking tips for pitta dosha

1. Cook food by using little spices, salt, or instant masalas (instant dhokla) as they preserve by using vinegar.
2. Use spices which are having cooling effect.
3. Use sweet fruits.
4. Use ghee, oil in adequate quantity.
5. Avoid new grains as it increases pitta, specially jaggery, wheat, rice, pulses.
6. Don't miss the food, take heavy breakfast.

Breakfast Menus for Pitta –

1. Start your morning with little warm water, you can add lemon to it.
2. Better to avoid tea coffee but if you want to take, make it low concentration by using less tea, coffee powder. Don't take too hot.
3. Milk can be preferred by adding cardamom.
4. Any juice, kadha can be taken like amla, guduchi, aloe vera.
5. You can use sweet semolina, upma, chapati – cooked vegetable, rice- daal moong laddu, groundnut chikki, kheer frequently.

6. For breakfast use moderately thalipeeth, poha, puri, sprouts .Food items with less oil, salt and spices.

7. Use rarely omelet, south Indian dishes like idly, dhokla, Vada, samosa.

Lunch Menu for Pitta Dosh Prakriti –

a. **Rotis** - Use chapatis with ghee. Wheat chapati is good. avoid Maida roti (tandoor, nan). Jowar is good for pitta. Bajra is hot irritating pitta better to use little.

b. **Vegetables** – cook vegetables by using low masalas. Sweet, astringent vegetables are good for pitta. Cabbage, cauliflower, sweet potatoes, potatoes are good for pitta.

1. Cabbage vegetable – it is good to balance pitta.

   Ingredients – 250 gm cabbage, salt, red chili or green chili, curry leaves, coriander, oil, mustard, cumin, onion, groundnut powder 2 tsp.

   Method – heat the pan, add oil, add mustard, cumin let it pop up, curry leaves, add chopped onion let it fry, add washed chopped cabbage, salt, chili, groundnut powder, cook for 5 minutes. garnish with coriander.

   This vegetable can be made by adding any pulse like moong, Toor, masoor for taste. This can be made by using tomatoes, green peas or besan.

2. French beans vegetable – good for pitta. can be made with same process.

3. Sweet potatoes -good for pitta, vata, increases kapha dosha.

   Ingredient- sweet potatoes 200 gm, oil, salt, red chili, coriander, mustard, cumin

Method – boil potatoes, heat the pan, add oil, mustard, cumin, let it pop up add chopped potatoes, other ingredients. Mix well cook for 3 minutes.

4. Carrots – carrots are good for pitta, use moderately in kapha. It can be made same as other vegetables like cabbage, cook well so becomes easy to digest. Carrots are used to make pickles, Murrumba, chutneys, kachumber, halva.

5. Onion vegetable – onion is used as a spice in Indian food culture. onion is good for vata pitta, increases kapha. It is used to make gravy's, masalas, kachumber's, it is eaten raw with spicy items, main ingredient of all chat like bhel, pani puri etc. onion vegetable can be made by frying with salt, chili. It can be used as side dish also.

6. Green vegetables – these are best used for pitta prakriti person. Spinach, wheat grass, zucchini is good for pitta, wash, cook with little spices.

7. Sprouts – sprouts are hard to digest according to ayurved literature but for change pitta can use with little spices. For making sprouts soak for 8 hours, change water, cook well with pressure cooker, then make with less oil, salt, chili.

8. Karela – bitter gourd – it is best for pitta, kapha, increases vata dosha. Karela juice, pickle, chutneys are famous.

   Ingredients – karela – 250 gm, onion, tamarind or lemon juice, turmeric, salt, red chili, coconut powder, groundnut powder – 1 tsp., oil, mustard, cumin,

   Method - wash karela, chop in round pieces, remove inner seeds (you can use with seeds also), heat the pan, add oil, cumin mustards, other ingredients, cook for 2 minutes, add karela, some water to cook. Cook for 5 minutes. You can make dry or little gravy as per your choice.

9. Radish – mooli- it should be used by cooking and low spices. parathas can be made with radish.

10. Lady's finger – it is favorite vegetable of children. available in all seasons.

Ingredients – lady's finger – 250 gm, onion, mustard, cumin, turmeric, groundnut powder, red chili, coconut powder, lemon juice 4 drops, salt, oil

Method – wash, dry for some time, cut as per your choice vertical, or round shape, heat the pan, add oil pop up mustard, cumin, add other ingredients, cook for 3 minutes, add lady's finger, cook for 5 minutes. Some people add curd, tomatoes for taste. We can make it as masala bhindi by filling bhindi with coconut, groundnut powder, salt, red chili, dhania powder. 2 tsp curd.

c. **Daal** – pulses – moong curry is best for pitta. Use Toor daal moderately. Masoor daal, chana daal moderately. Bengal gram (chole), black gram (urad daal) hoarse gram (kulthi)is pitta irritating so use very little.

d. **Rice –**

basmati, white, shashtishali (homemade – direct from farm without polishing) rice is good for pitta. avoid brown rice. plain rice with ghee is good for pitta. While making pulao, biryani use little masalas.

e. **Papad** – moong papad is good for pitta, but as papad is by adding spices salts, pitta should use little. Other papad like urad, small millet is pitta irritating. Rice papad can be used moderately. potato papad moderately.

f. **Pickles** – as most of pickles are pitta irritating better to use occasionally. Sweet pickles of mango, lemon, amla, haldi in moderate is good for pitta.

g. **Salads** – salads or raitas are good for pitta as they are having adequate water content. Especially cucumber, carrots, are good for pitta. Other cabbage, tomato's, beet can be used moderately.

Use fresh curd for raitas, better to use in afternoon lunch.

h. – **chutneys** – pitta can use chutneys moderate like groundnut, mix daal. coconut is good for pitta so can use daily, it will nourish pitta and best cooling agent. Avoid sesame as it is pitta irritating.

i. **beverages** – buttermilk is best for pitta by adding salt or sugar, cumin powder. Curd with sugar is good for pitta.

Evening snacks – as pitta is having a glutton habit, he needs evening snacks. prefer tea coffee only in winter, rainy seasons. Mint tea or kadha made up of ginger, honey, guduchi is good for pitta. any sweet fruit can be taken like sweet apple, grapes, pomegranate, banana, mangoes, watermelon, sugarcane (juice). other items which are available like rice, chapati, laddu (moong, coconut, rajgira,), homemade snacks (chivda, Shankar Pala, chikki) but made it by using wheat flour. Better to avoid besan products or use little.

Soaked nuts like almonds, raisins, figs, deserts made up of dates, dates soaked in ghee can be used as pitta needs nourishment. Any fruit juice, lassi, mattha, coconut water good for pitta.

Dinner menus for pitta prakruti –

Better to take dinner earlier at 7 pm. You can use chapati daal, cooked vegetables, rice soups in dinner. Any homemade desert like kheer, halva, sweet rotis are good for pitta.

Milk with turmeric if tolerated can be taken before going to bed, some pitta people may have loose stool due to milk so prefer as you tolerate.

Hoteling for pitta prakriti – pitta prakriti person prefer clean, neat hotels with fair prices. Better to avoid Chinese, Mexican, spicy, salty food. simple food items are well tolerated by pitta instead of fancy foods. Prefer dry cooling light food. Follow regular rules as given above. Mix vegetable soup, beans soup, mocktails can be used. Avoid using too much combinations of food.

Pitta vata prakriti – follow all the rules of pitta as pitta is predominant but take care for vata. Pitta needs cooling agents but as vata may irritate use warm. warm water, warm deserts are preferred.

- **Breakfast-** warm milk, warm water with lemon, aloe vera juice, milk with cardamom, milk with turmeric, milk with ginger, mint tea
- Sweet semolina, upma (less spicy), kheer, sweet roti, chapati – cooked vegetables, rice – daal, parathas (carrot, cabbage, potato), sweet puri. For change can use rice flakes, idly, Dosa, moong chilla, laddus (moong, wheat flour, rice)
- **Lunch** – wheat flour chapati with ghee, any cooked vegetable (less spicy), plain rice, daal (moong), use moderately Toor daal, masoor daal. Buttermilk with sugar, salt, curd, cooked salads, sweet pickles, moong papad, are good for pitta vata.

Snacks - sweet puri, wheat flour laddu, sugarcane juice, mango juice, plain dosa, kheer, sweet roti (Dashami)

Dinner – chapati, less spicy curry or cooked vegetable, rice with ghee, fresh kadhi, khichari, daal rice.

Pitta kapha prakriti Diet plan –

For pitta kapha plan priory for pitta but care for kapha. Diet which are moderately warm soft but little dry are preferred for both dosha. Deserts are good for pitta but as kapha is secondary take moderately warm deserts with less sugar. Manage owing to your Agni, because pitta having strong fire, kapha low.

Breakfast – warm milk with cardamon, warm water with honey, lemon, mint tea, chapati cooked vegetable, daal rice, paratha with less ghee, rarely use idly, poha, upma, less spicy puri, mint chutney.

Lunch – chapati or fulka a is good, cooked vegetables, mint coriander chutney, cabbage, cauliflower

C. Kapha Dosh Prakriti

As kapha is unctuous, oily, slimy, sticky so kapha may use dry, light, hot food

Key points – dry, light, hot, eat when hungry and drink when thirsty is the golden rule for kapha.

General rules for kapha –

1. Cook food with lots of spices for kapha as they are having low stomach fire (fenugreek, cumin, turmeric).
2. meals are sufficient for kapha.
3. snacking between meal is avoided as kapha digest food slowly.
4. fasting is good for kapha.
5. don't use food for emotions (avoid emotional eating) like biscuits, chocolates, ice-cream.
6. frozen cold food not good for kapha
7. kapha should avoid heavy, oily food. food with low calorie, low fat is good for kapha.
8. food should be cooked by dry methods like baking, sautéing, grilling rather than boiling, cooking.
9. use little oil or ghee for kapha.

Breakfast – warm water, kadha (Tulsi, ginger, black pepper, jaggery, clove), mint tea, lemon water is good for kapha. Phulka – vegetable, Methi paratha, moong chili, upma, is good for kapha.

1. Kadha / green tea/ herbal tea/ mint tea/ginger tea are good options for kapha.
2. Moong chila – moong chila is best menu for kapha, pitta.

Ingredients – moong 200 gm, green chili 2-3, salt, cumin powder, oil, coriander

Method – soak moong for 2 hours, grind in mixer make batter add salt, grinded chili other ingredients in it. Mix well, heat pan (Dosa tava),put some oil, add batter spread with spreader,cook for 3 minutes and serve with mint chutney.

3. Methi Paratha (Thepla)- Methi paratha is best for kapha dosha .

Ingredients – Methi 200 gm, wheat flour 250 gm, salt, coriander, dhania powder, sesame seeds, red chili, oil

Method – wash Methi cook for 2 minutes to make it soft, now make dove by adding all ingredients. make bolls, roll by roti roller and roast with pan. serve with mint chutney, pickle, curd.

3. Upma – semolina upma occasional use is good for kapha.
4. Sandwich – bread or bakery items are not recommended in ayurved but you can use once in a month for change. Kapha can use toasts as they are airy.

Lunch menus for kapha –

1. **Chapatis / rotis** – as wheat are kapha vitiating, use occasionally, phulkas are good for kapha, without ghee or oil. Jowar roti (millet) are better to use. Can Use small millet (bajara) moderately.
2. **Vegetables** – fresh cooked vegetables are good for kapha
3. Beet, cabbage, cauliflower, carrot, drumstick, fenugreek is good for kapha. Avoid potato, tomato, paneer, curd, cheese, milk products.
4. **Curry's** – moong daal is best for kapha. Red gram, Bengal gram, red lentils are also beneficial for kapha.
5. **Pickles** – kapha can use pickles moderately. as it is good for kapha.
6. **Chutneys** – mint, garlic, amla chutney are good for kapha. Avoid coriander, coconut chutneys. Dry chutneys are good then wet to balance kapha.
7. **Rice** – rice is sweet, kapha irritating, better to take moderately. It is best to roast rice and use. avoid new grain, at least keep for 6-8 months.
8. **Kachumber** – raitas' – use carrots, onion, beets for making kachumber. use fresh curd for raita, but use occasionally.
9. **Papad** – moong, red gram papad are used, best to eat by roasting, avoid fry papad. Avoid. urad, rice papad.

10. **Dairy products** – low calorie dairy products are preferred. Add water in milk, buttermilk with salt or trikatu is good for kapha. Panner, cheese, better to avoid.

11. **Sweet** – deserts – as kapha dosha is already sweet use occasional deserts. strictly avoid deserts at night as they are heavy and had to digest. Deserts can be made by adding less sugar. Better to use old jaggery. Chikkis, groundnut laddus, sweet semolina (less ghee, sugar), gudroti, sweet roti of sesame is best to use.

12. **Buttermilk / Peya** – kapha can use fresh buttermilk by adding spices like cumin powder, saindhav.

13. **Soups** – soups are good for kapha to stimulate stomach fire or for easy digestion. Mix vegetables, corn, mushroom soups are good for kapha.

Evening snacks – the golden rule for kapha is eat when hungry and drink when thirsty so usually kapha doesn't require any evening snack. but if needed can take any fruit like, pomegranate, guava, papaya, coconut water, sugarcane juice, nimbu pani, laja, roasted chana, cucumber.

Dinner – kapha should take light dinner before 7 pm for good digestion. Heavy, spicy, sweet dinner should be strictly avoided.

Menus –

1. Phulka – without oil, ghee. better to use jowar (millet) roti.
2. Vegetables -fenugreek, drumstick, cabbage, cauliflower are good to use with less oil, can use spice moderately.
3. Rice – khichari, plain rice, daal khichari can be taken in small quantity. Rice should be old. For khichari moong daal is good.
4. Soups – kapha can use soups of various vegetables abundantly. Better in evening if they can take only soups with one phulka.

Eating out (hoteling) for kapha dosha –

Kapha must use warm water or better if he carries his own water. Eat warm cooked food, avoid spicy, oily, creamy, sweet deserts. Start with any vegetable soup without cream. Tandoor roti is ok for kapha. Naan, butter naan, kulcha will be heavy to digest. Use warm deserts if necessary. Steamed salads, little spicy vegetable, plain rice- daal is good for kapha. Occasional use of Chinese, Indian continental food is ok. avoid Mexican, Italian food as it may be prepared with creamy dressing, Maida, butter etc. Avoid cakes, pastry's, pudding's, cold water, ice-creams etc.

Little wine or bear is ok for kapha prakriti. use tambool or paan for mukhshudhdi. Better to take light diet for next day.

Diet for Dwidoshaj prakriti dual constitution

1. **Kaph-vata prakriti** – as kapha is dominant person can follow all kapha recipes.

Breakfast – Ginger tea, jaggery tea, warm milk with cardamom, lemongrass tea, warm water

Other menu- spicy upma, spicy semolina, chapati- cooked vegetable, daal rice

Lunch – chapati - phulka, cabbage, cauliflower, lady's finger, curry, mix salad (steamed), rice, pickles can be used, chutneys

Evening snacks – hot milk with cinnamon, laja, chivda, any fruit, tea,

Dinner – mix vegetable soup, phulka, cooked vegetable, khichari, fresh kadhi, spinach vegetable,

2. **Kapha – pitta prakriti-** diet which is described for kapha can be used but as pitta is secondary avoid too much hot, spices warm is good for both dosha.

Breakfast – warm milk with cardamon, warm milk with haldi, semolina less spicy, thalipeeth, idly (occasionally)

Lunch – phulka with cooked vegetables karela, Methi, Shepu can be used. Fresh buttermilk with saindhav, steamed salad (carrot, cucumber, beet).

Afternoon – mint tea, laja, oats, Raggi, chivda, seasonal fruit,

Dinner – khichari (vegetable Pulao) with kadhi, jowar roti – cooked vegetables, moong daal khichari.

Chapter 5

Veg – Nonveg Diet

What to eat vegetarian or nonvegetarian it is choice or right of human to select his own food. according to ayurveda classical references vegetarian diet (shakahar) is mostly classified in various Vargas . all Nighantus also classified food types like shhak varg, phal varg, vari varg etc. detailed description of this classification is available in classics.

Acharya charka has elaborated all details in Annapanavidhi Adhyaya. but very less indications are given about nonvegetarian diet.

In Jwara (fever), Rajkshyama (Tuberculosis), shosh (debility) Mamrasa (meat soup) is indicated. Meat soup Basti (enema) is indicated in Asthi majja (bone- bone marrow) disorders. Even in seasonal regimen acharya indicated quantity of meat, which meat is good to eat etc.

As per anatomy or physiology considered humans teeth are likely to use to chew food not to tear food. But some animals have sharp teeth, nails. These animal secrete more acid for digestion, length of intestine is equal to body (so food easily passes through gastrointestinal tract) but as humans have lengthy intestinal track .

Vegetarian diet	non-vegetarian diet
Vegetarian diet helps to increase sattva attribute. it is preferred during rituals, Indian festivals.	It influences raja & tama attributes.
we get of second class proteins from veg diet but in sufficient quantity. Vegetarian diet contains carbohydrates & minerals.	First class proteins are available in non-vegetarian diet.
Veg diet contains Roughage makes food easy to digest	Very less roughage heavy to digest may cause constipation
Variety of food available	As compared variety is few.
Vitamin b_{12} less available but can be taken from milk products	Good amount of vitamin b 12 is available
Calcium is available in milk products.	Calcium is available in good quantity
Chances are moderate to gain weight	Effectively gains weight due to regular consumption.
Food can be stored for long	Food preservation required for long storage.
Less chances for infection through food	Infection Chances increases

if health or diseases are considered as per research studied nonvegetarian people may suffer from cardiovascular diseases like hypertension, angina, atherosclerosis. weight gain, hemorrhoids, constipation, are some common problems observed in nonvegetarian people. it is due to high presence of fats proteins, cholesterol in it .

vegetarian diet gives more satiety, increase oja, satvikata (mindfulness), resistance power on the other hand nonveg diet raises Tama raja Guna which creates violence.

Chapter 6

Incompatible diet – Virodhi Ahara

The food which is having adverse effect on metabolism, digestion, circulation is called as incompatible diet. The concept of incompatible diet is well explained by our Acharya's. such type of food causes various problems like indigestion, poor absorption, blockage of channel's, development of Ama.

Acharya charka clearly states that the food which aggravates dosha is viruddh Ahara. Viruddha Ahara is the main causative factor for skin problems, metabolic diseases, indigestion.

Visham Bhojan – the food which keep balance in normal (prakruti) dosha, and normalize imbalanced dosha into normal is hitkar (beneficial) Ahara. The food in combinations, opposite attributes, unfavorable conditions may cause diseases.

Types of Visham bhojan –

1. Adhyashan – to take food before digestion of earlier food is not recommended in ayurveda. Food should be taken after digestion of earlier food.
2. Vishamasan – to take food in any time like late night, early morning. Food should be consumed on proper time.

3. Samashan – to take wholesome & unwholesome food combinedly it causes tridosh aggravation.
4. Anashan – fasting – continuous fasting leads to malnutrition, complexion reduction, constipation, debility, disturbed mind. Acharya charka has elaborated incompatible diet in following way.

Dietetic incompatibility

a. **Desha viruddha** – intake of food / diet with similar attributes of that particular Desha (region). For example, persons from Anupa Desh (moisture, unctuous) should not consume moist, unctuous food, this will be contraindicatory. dry region – dry food not recommended.

b. **Kala viruddha** – diet contradicted to specific season, time. To eat sheet (cold), Ruksha (dry) food in winter. To eat Ushna (hot), tikshna (spicy) food in summer.

c. **Agni viruddha** – diet which is not accordingly one's digestive fire. Consuming laghu (light), Ruksha (dry) food when Agni is high (teekshnagni – high digestive fire). Consuming guru (heavy) diet when Agni is mand (slow digestive fire).

d. **Matra viruddha** – intake of diet which is incompatible as per quantity. food should be consumed accordingly quantity – intake of ghee & honey in equal quantity.

e. **Satmya viruddha** – intake of food which is not suitable to that person, for example the person who takes soft, simple food suddenly he changed food habits with hot pungent. The person who never takes any beverages if he consumes beverages like alcohol, coca cola.

f. **Dosh viruddha** – diet which is contraindicated to that person is called as dosha viruddha. for kapha prakriti sheet (cold), guru (heavy), Madhur (sweet) food is not recommended it will aggravate kapha dosha.

g. **Sanskar viruddha** – method of preparing food items or what process is applied for cooking food. Curd is not cooked, heated honey, peacock meat cooked in castor oil.

h. **Virya viruddha** – sheet (cold) & Ushna (hot) food combined not recommended or contraindicated it is said to be virya viruddha. Milk and horse gram – milk is cold and horse gram are hot in potency. Some more combinations are like milk and meat, milk and yogurt, milk, and sour fruits

i. **Koshth viruddha** – intake of food which is contraindicated to koshth (nature of intestine). intake of hot, spicy heavy food person with mrudu koshth (soft bowl) is not recommended. Same way dry, light food consumption by krura koshth (dry bowl).

j. **Avastha viruddha** – food contraindicated with one's physical & diseased status. The person who gets daily sun exposure eats hot spicy food which is contraindicated. Guru (heavy) bhojan in Jwara (fever), Atisar (diarrhea), laghu bhojan in debility, sheet (cold) food in cough & cold.

k. **Parihar viruddha** – the food which is contraindicated accordingly sequence. After abhyanga (olation) drinking of cold water which is not recommended it causes blockages (strotoavrodh). Intake of heavy food after Vamana, Basti. intake of water before tea.

l. **Paak viruddha** – food which is unevenly or improperly cooked in contraindicated. It may be food which is burned, overcooked, overheated food.

m. **Samyoga viruddha** – food which is not supposed to combine with each other. Sour fruits and milk both are having different potency (banana milkshake, strawberry milkshake) yogurt with meat.

n. **Hrut viruddha** – food which is not pleasant to that person. It may be having variety as per persons choice.

o. **Sampad viruddha** – food which is not made by using proper qualities such food is contraindicated. food or fruits which are not having proper taste, color, over ripened, stale food. Meat of diseased animal, Sheera (sweet semolina) prepared in vegetable oil (Dalda).

p. **Upchar viruddha** – the food which is contraindicated after specific act or upchar (treatment). Drinking cold water, drinks, beverages after Sneha, intake of guru Ahar after Vamana, intake of guru Ahar, Madhur bhojan after Virechana

Some 21ˢᵗ Century's Incompatible Diet

1. Sweets with Alcohol – fat saturation
2. Juice and Dalia – blood sugar tolls
3. Fried meat, eggs – load to digest as high protein
4. Cheese and Beans – apposite properties
5. Cold Water with food – lowers stomach fire
6. Fries, Pizzas with Coke
7. Cola and fries – apposite property
8. Fruits with Yogurt - apposite properties
9. Fruits after Meals- apposite properties
10. Mixed Vegetables like kaju - Paneer, Malai- Palak,
11. Juice and Cereal - apposite properties
12. Curd Chicken - apposite properties
13. Tea & Milk - apposite properties
14. Drinking water before tea or after tea or hot beverages
15. samosa and tea - apposite properties
16. pizza and coke - apposite properties

chapter 7

Important Food Items

A. Grains – Shali Dhanya

1. **Rice** – rice is main food (first food) for millions of people. rice has been used from decades as a main source of energy, even for childhood it is highly favoured food. almost in all states of India first food of baby is rice.

   rice is not only used as a food but it is having a great contribution in holy festivals, pooja, marriages, welcome ceremony. in pooja rice are used as in ayurveda rice is classified in four categories.

   1. Shali – it is preferred in winter season 2. Raktshali – red in colour preferred for all, nutritious
   2. Vrihi- grows during rainy season
   3. Shashtik – it grows in sixty days.
      rice is available in hundreds of varieties, in every state different type of rice has been used.

      it has various types according to quality, colour, shape, growing period etc.

some famous varieties of rice are as below

- a. basmati - according to ayurved basmati are good for all dosha. these are used for preparing variety of dishes. elongated,
- b. Indrayani – little big but tastes good.
- c. Kolam – preferred much for daily purpose.
- d. Hmt – preferred mostly.
- e. Chinnor – flavoured rice variety earlier around 25 yrs. back red rice or farm made rice (without processing) preferred for routine use. but now a days people prefer white and polished rice.

rice is good source of carbohydrate, protein according to ayurved it sweet, nourishes dhatus. it is best for vata, pitta dosha and it increases kapha dosha. it is great source of vitamin b

old rice (6- 8 months long) good for use as new rice is heavy to digest and it creates ama . use new rice by roasting to avoid bad effects. rice prepared by roasting is good for patients as it becomes easy to digest.

don't wash rice too much as vitamins drain out by over – washing. using legumes with rice (daal- rice) best balancing dish for vitamin b12.

in andhra pradesh, goa,kokan, karnatak rice is main meal and people can stay on rice only. rice water (tanduloka) is best source of minerals,best for skin,hair, taken along with medicine as anupana.

2. **Wheat** – wheat is widely used for making roti, chapati, puri, phulka, laddus in India.

wheat flour is made by grinding wheat. wheat is great source of proteins. vitamins, specially cover of wheat is rich in fibres. whole wheat flour is good for good digestion. wheat flour is also known as atta, chakki, chakki atta or chapati atta. Wheat is available in various variety like sharbati, Panjabi etc.

plain wheat roti is good for vata, pitta dosha, kapha should use without ghee or oil.

3. **Jowar**- Millets – (white millet) – jowar is also known as jondhala, jwarrie. Along with wheat it is widely used in India in main meal. jowar roti – besan, jowar roti – bharta is the famous food. jowar is thick and oily then wheat so oil is not required for making roti. In winter season it is made by applying sesame seeds. Jowar roti is light and easy to digest. it is best for tridosha. In Maharashtra many people jowar roti instead of wheat as it is good for overall nourishment.

4. **Bajara** – Black Millet – bajara is dry, hot so best for kapha prakriti. bajara flour is light grey in colour. Due to dry property not much recommended for vata, pitta. Bajara roti with ghee is mostly used in winter which is best for nourishment.

5. **Nachani** - finger millet - ragi or Nachani flour is best option for every age. it is great source of minerals, calcium and fibre. Nachani is best for kapha if used excess increases vata and pitta dosha. Nachani can be used for making roti, Papad, dosa. As ragi is light dry, warming it is best used for kapha disorders. Ragi flour In various combinations used to improve digestion, agnimandya (low stomach fire), Aam, obesity, cholesterol. As it is sattvic if less oil is used it can be used for tridosha. It is best food for new-born babies.

6. **Satu** – – Satu is made by roasted chana and wheat flour. it best used in summer due to its cooling effect. Satu is mainly used in north region as food. In Panjab it is used in sharbat form. Satu is best for pitta pacification.

7. **Corn** – variety of Corn is available in India. sweet corn, baby corn, American corn. corn can be used half boiled or baked with spices, oil salt. In rainy season mostly corn is preferred by baking with salt and masala. Some people use Maka roti as a main meal. in Panjab maka roti with sarso sabji is the famous traditional dish in winter. Maka is preferred for constipation. it balances pitta, kapha

but irritates vata dosha. Maka is best used with milk. Corn can be widely used as to make Corn soup, corn pakora, corn paratha, corn vade. Corn flakes are used with milk as breakfast menu.

8. **Singadha** – water walnut - it is available from water resources. It is used fresh, dry or boiled. mostly singadha is used during fast. singadha roti is famous dish during fast. dried powder of singadha is used for various dishes like roti, kheer, puri. acharya charka explained in detail about medicinal properties of singadha in infertility, pitta disorders, shukravruddhi (Aphrodisiac), repeated abortions, diarrhoea etc. due to its Madhur property pacifies pitta dosha.

9. **Rajgira** – Amaranthus – it is used as cereal and vegetable also. Sweet in taste and having pungent potency. Leafy vegetable is used with roti. As a cereal dried powder is used to make roti. It is widely used during fast. it is a great source of proteins and minerals. Acharya charka mentioned Amaranthus in vegetable class (shak varg), Marisha is the Sanskrit name . this is available in two varieties swetha and rakta maarisha .it balance pitta dosha and best used in pitta Vikara.

A. Pulses –

As we have discussed main cereals, mostly cereals are used with pulses in Indian culture. As rice Daal, chapati – vegetable. for rice mostly toor daal (pigeon pea) is used. moong, chana, masoor daal is used widely for making daal . pulses are great source of proteins.

Moong, masoor, Toor all types of Daal (soup of pulses) are used by boiling with water and adding rock salt, ginger, asafoetida etc to make it tasty and digestible. Actually, in ayurved all types of Daal are dry, sheet and vishtambhi so irritates vata dosha, to avoid this Daals can be used by adding oil, ghee and spices.

1. **Toor Daal** (pigeon pea) - in ayurved it is named as adhaki, tuvarak which is ruksha, Madhur, after digestion it becomes sweet. It is little heavy then other Daal it increase vata dosha and balances

pitta dosha. In Indian kitchen it is daily used to make daal, sambhar sabji. Daal is best used with ghee. it helps in treatment of poisoning, skin diseases

2. **Moong Daal** (green gram) – moong daal or green gram is widely used as it is best diet during panchakarma, very easy to digest. Sweet in taste, light and pungent in potency it nourishes all dhatus, varnya, good for eyes. In Gujrat yellow khichari is famous dish in all season as it nourishes sapta dhatu. Green gram is used to make regular Daal, sabji, Dosa, pakora, soup, Papad . Moong soup is famous and accepted dish for low stomach fire, after panchakarma, during treatment plan, to strengthen body tissue and to replenish.

3. **Chana Daal** (Bengal gram – chick pea)- it is also known as chanak, chole. It is used by steaming, boiling, frying powder form. This Daal is widely used for making various dishes like besan, bhaji, sabji, laddu, pakora etc. It vitiates vata dosha, balances pitta and kapha dosha. Ayurved acharyas explained detail properties of chana daal as boiled chana Daal gives strength, improves taste, steamed chickpea balances kapha pitta. Roasted chick pea are laghu, amahar, kledhar, adra chanak improves taste . chick pea soup is best for reduces excess kapha. Roasted salted chana daal is favourite snack of many people but it is too dry and irritates vata dosha.

4. **Masoor** – legumes – masoor is mainly used in north India for making Daal. It vitiates vata dosha and balances kapha, pitta. it is used in pitta vikar. masoor dry powder is widely used as a face pack ingredient. Masoor powder pack increases skin's beauty, it can be used by adding water or milk.

5. **Kulthi** – black gram - astringent taste, hot potency, dry, light in nature. Owing to its properties kulith pacifies kapha - vata dosha and irritates pitta rakta.

6. Kulthi soup or Daal is used in obese person, it is used as scrub in excess sweating. Kulthi soup is used in white discharge, scanty menses in women. As it decreases Shukra dhatu use is contraindicated in infertility patients.

7. **Chavali** – cowpea – in ayurved it is also known as rajmash, it is a rich source of proteins. it is available in various colours like reddish, white, black. It used as veggie or usal. sweet, dry, heavy to digest. It irritates vata dosha, balances kapha, pitta. It nourishes dhatu, increases quantity of stool, improves breast milk.

8. **Matar** – pea, field pea – in ayurved text it is named as kalaya. Dry sweet, cold in potency. It irritates vata dosha and balances pitta kapha. It is not recommended in vata vikar.

9. **Pavate** – beans – flat beans – dry light irritates vata dosha. it is used as veggie and usal.

10. **Soyabean** – tofu -now a days soya products are very famous rich source of proteins. In traditional ayurved soyabean was not included but now it is consumed very much. Soyabean is used in the form of oil, chunks, milk, nuts . due to phytoestrogen it is beneficial for vata constitution and vata dosha specially in women's during menopause, but irritates pitta kapha . in Maharashtra soyabean is used with regular wheat flower. It lowers cholesterol level. It helps in restoring health of heart. It is hard to digest sometimes it may cause constipation or diarrhoea. Always use soyabean by soaking overnight, cooking with spices.

B. Vegetables

Vegetables are best source of minerals and vitamins. In India most of people uses vegetables as a main meal with chapati or roti. Region wise different variety of Vegetables are available. as per the weather conditions different vegetables are available like in rainy season, winter or summer season. Some vegetables like carrot, cucumber, beet can be eaten raw, some by steaming, some by boiling.

Some common tips for using vegetables

1. Use fresh seasonal vegetables.
2. Wash well before use.
3. In rainy season use medicated or hot water for washing.

4. Cut in large pieces, before use. Don't put cute vegetables in refrigerator
5. Use little water for leafy vegetable.
6. Cook on low flame, for a while. don't cook for long as cooking losses nutritious values.
7. Add salt at the end of cooking it enhances digestion.

Vegetables are categorised under

1. leafy & nonleafy vegetables.
2. Raw & cooked vegetables

1. Nonleafy vegetables

a. **Tomato** – tomatoes are best source of vitamin A, B, C, iron . tomatoes are widely used for veggies, soup, puri, chat ani, pickle etc. sweet sour in taste increases all three doshas.

b. **Potato** – potatoes are transported from Europe to India. Sweet, salty in rasa cool potency. Irritates vata, pacifies pitta & kapha dosha. Potatoes widely used for making various dishes like veggie, paratha, wafers, chat, Papad, potatoes are favourite for children. cook potatoes with cover, don't peel of before cooking.

c. **Onion** – onions are soul of Indian kitchen. It is used as a spice and for various purposes. Sweet pungent, guru, snigdh, sweet potency. Balances vata, slightly increase kapha. Onions are aphrodisiac in nature, promotes strength. According to ayurved onions are rajasic in nature. onions are available in pink and white colour.

d. **Carrot** – carrots are good source of vitamin A. sweet, bitter, balances vata pitta dosha. Carrots are used as veggie, halva, pickles. Carrot halva is famous dish in winter season. It nourishes dhatu. Promotes digestion.

e. **Cucumber** – cucumber is great source of water, balances water. Sweet, light, cold potency, pitta pacifying, neutral. Used for burning sensations. eating raw cucumber is wrong as it irritates vata dosha. Mostly people prefer cucumber as a salad. it is best to use cucumber by little steaming with ghee and rock salt. It is used for veggies, paratha. Avoid eating during rainy season, best to use in winter and summer.

f. **Beet** – beet is sweet in taste, ushna virya balances vata dosha, may increase pitta and kapha. Beets are good source of vitamins and minerals. Can be used to treat constipation, anaemia.

g. **Garlic** – garlic is pungent, ushna virya increases pitta, balances kapha vata. garlic is used as spice in Indian kitchen. Due to its ushna pungent it is used to balance vata and kapha vikar. Vata and kapha prakriti people must include garlic in diet.

h. **lady's finger** – bhindi – sweet, cold balances vata pitta, vitiates kapha dosha. It is a famous vegetable. it is used in diabetes, urinary infections.

i. **Cabbage** – sweet astringent, balances kapha, pitta irritates vata dosha. It is good source of fibres, vitamin, minerals. It is used in veggie, paratha, salad, Chinese dishes.

j. **Cauliflower** – astringent, cool, irritates vata, balances pitta and kapha. It is best to treat constipation.

k. **Radish** – pungent, bitter, light, balances three dosha. Radish is used as salad, veggie, Parathas. It is use to make shandaki and kanjika. it is best to use radish in piles, pain, throat infection.

l. **Surana** – jimikand – elephant foot – astringent, pungent, laghu, ruksh . pacifies kapha vata.

m. **Lauki** – bottle gourd – bitter, light, vata pitta dosha. Lauki is used in veggies, paratha, puddings, kheer, halva, laddu. according to classics it is vamak, not good for hrdya. So, use little in children, pregnant and old age person. It is cooling light, easy to digest.

n. **Drumstick** – shigru – pungent, bitter, balances kapha vata

o. **Brinjal** – baingan – baingan sabji or bharta is traditional dish in Maharashtra prepared during festival of gauri poojan . sweet, ushna in nature, balances vata kapha little increase of pitta dosha. As per Nighantu it increases kapha, pitta, as the studies or tradition it is avoided in skin diseases. It is shukral (aphrodisiac) best to use in amavata (rheumatoid arthritis).

Brinjal is used with rice, as veggie, chutney, fried pieces are good Appetizer. White brinjal are good for haemorrhoids. Brinjal must be used by cooking as it contains alkali and vitamins. Roasted brinjal are best for kapha vata pacification.

p. **Ridge gourd** – koshtaki – Dodki, Turai, Gilki – bitter, pungent, light, dry, pacifies kaph pitta and increases vata dosha. As it is vamak in nature used before panchakarma as a vamak (emetic) drug.

q. **Chilli's –** red chilis – or mirchi is main spice in Indian kitchen. Pungent, dry, strong, hot in potency. Pacifies kapha vata and irritates pitta dosha. Excess use cause irritation of stomach, burning sensation, thirst, diarrhoea. Chillies are used for its pungent taste for making various dishes. Green chillies are also used in kitchen as a spice, especially for making poha, upma, thecha, green chutney, kadhi etc. Green chilis are dried and fine powder is used in Indian kitchen. As a custom Indian women make red chili powder for whole year.

r. **Ghevada** - broad beans – good source of protein, vitamin. These are used by cooking or steaming with masala for better digestion. These beans are good for vata dosha making with masala.

s. **Farasbi** – French beans - French bean sabji is great source of energy and tastes good . it can be used with roti, chapati, bread.–

t. **Nimbu** – lemon - nimbu is a versatile item widely used for various purposes as food, medicine or for making medicines . unripe lemon it is sour, little pungent balances vata, kapha, increases pitta. Ripe lemon balances pitta and kapha. Lemon is used as side menu with lunch,dinner. 3-4 drops of lemon in sabji, daal,rice, poha, upma, or spicy dish makes it more tastier and healthier. Lemon juice is good appetizer, carminative, digestive substance. Lemon pickle are preferred during low stomach fire or indigestion. Nimbu sharbat is all time favourite, all-purpose drink which gives quick energy. It is preferred during fasting, diarrhoea, vomiting, indigestion to balance fluid levels. Sour lemon pickle are good for vata and sweet lemon pickle is good for pitta dosha. Lemon is used for purification of metals while making medicines. Lemons are good toner for skin and hair used as antibiotic, antibacterial, antifungal substance.

u. **Kadhipatta** – curry leaves – kaidarya- curry leaves are used for flavours or decoration as its fragrance is stimulating and exciting. Curry leaves are used in Daal, sabji, chutney, poha, upma, sambar, masala rice, pulao etc. they are pungent, bitter in nature balances kapha, vata increases pitta dosha. It is good carminative, digestive, appetizer agent. Chewing curry leaves or boiling with water maintains health.

v. **Simla mirchi** – capsicum – it is available in colours like red, green, yellow. Capsicums are good source of energy aggravate vata and pitta dosha. They are used as mild spice. Used in Chinese snacks like noodles, pizza. In India it is used for sabji, pav- bhaji, veg roll, chutney.

w. **Padval** – snake gourd – patol – it is bitter, pungent, light, dry balances kapha and pitta dosha. In ayurved patol is used as amapachak for various toxic conditions. Used to improve digestion, liver disease, fever.

x. **Ghosali** – smooth gourd – Bimbi - these are small bitter, light, small balances kapha pitta, increases vata dosha. In Maharashtra specially they are used for making pakora, sabji. nutritionally good excess use is contraindicated as they are vamak (emetic).

y. **Gavar** – cluster beans – gavar balances pitta and irritates vata, kapha dosha. Gavar is used by little steaming or boiling. Gavar sabji made with spices help to balance three dosha.

2 Leafy - Green vegetables –

Though green vegetables are composed of less nutrients compared to other one, but they are required for better health. green vegetables are full of fibres, roughage, iron and minerals. nonvegetarian people may include in their diet. green vegetables are mostly used for stuffing like paratha, bhaji,

Vada, kabab. Green vegetables are good source of iron specially spinach, dhania, Rajgira etc.

Fresh Green vegetables are good to use if not available some use dried powder. You can store green vegetables by drying.

1. **Spinach** – palak – available for whole year. Great source of iron, calcium, minerals, vitamins. Pungent, sweet, cold, may increase vata, kapha dosha. Palak is heavy to digest. Milk should be avoided with green vegetables. Palak is used with Daal (Daal-palak),paratha, bhaji, pakora, veggie,as stuff for chats. better to use by steaming

2. **Methika** – fenugreek – bitter, pungent, light hot potency, good for vata and pitta little increase in pitta. It is great source of vitamins and used as katupoushtik for puerperal women as it stimulates breast milk. It is good for children's, pregnant women for strength and nourishment. Fenugreek seeds are used for external and internal application. It is good for hair, skin, digestion, urinary infection, lowers cholesterol.

   Methika is used as veggie, for making laddu, paratha.

3. **Shepu** – Dill seeds – shatpushpa, shatava – bitter, pungent, vata kapha balancing, irritates pitta dosha. It is a good source of iron and vitamins. Shatapushpa is very beneficial for women. Many use shepu and palak together for making sabji. it is best for puerperal women's is a natural aphrodisiac.

4. **Chuka** – bladder dog (green sorrel) – sour, sweet, light, hot potency. Balances vata and irritates pitta and kapha dosha. Improves digestion. it is used with Daal, as veggie

5. **Dhania** – coriander – Dhanyak – astringent, bitter, light, sweet, hot potency, balances three dosha. Coriander drink is very easy to make best for reducing thirst in summer. In Indian kitchen coriander is having great importance as it is used for garnishing the dishes. It is used for making chutney, Vada, parathas, it improves

taste and looks good. seeds, leaves, fruit is used for medicinal purpose.

6. **Kardi** – kusumb, safflower – pungent, heavy, hot, strong, hot potency increases tridosha. In some texts it is described as kapha pacification. Safflower oil is widely used for cooking.

7. **Tandulja** – Chinese spinach - sweet, cold potency, dry light, balances kapha and pitta dosha. Mostly it is used as veggie with rotis. Available tribal areas of India.

8. **Ambadi** – basterd jute (Gonjura leaves) – it is best source of iron, folic acid. In different it known as different names. Widely used in India, available in tribal areas. Ambadi sabji and roti is the famous dish in Maharashtra.

9. **Aluchi pane** – green taro – arbi patra- pungent, bitter, hot, light. it is good source of calcium, iron. Used as a neurotronic, juice is used for wound healing. It is good for general health. Leaf's are used for making vadi (Alu vadi) which is famous in Maharashtra.

10. **Rajgira** – Amaranthus – Marisha -sweet heavy pungent in nature, slightly increases dosha. Balances pitta dosha, increases vata, kapha. Two varieties are available. Rajgira seeds are nutritionally good used during fasting. Great source of minerals, calcium you can consume seeds with milk. Rajgira laddu, chikki, rotis are preferred in Navratri fasting.

11. **Math** – red math – Red Amaranthus – rich source of fibre and nutritious. available all over India. it is made by little steaming.

12. **Harbhara** – chana leaves – astringent dry, cold. Increases Vata, balances pitta kapha. Chanak leaves are used as veggie in tribal areas of India. It stimulates stomach fire.

13. **Hadga** – available in tribal area. Used by steaming in little oil, tastes good with jowar roti.

14. **Takla** - available in tribal area, nutritious.

15. **Kurdu** – available in tribal area and in rainy season.

16. **Kanda paat** – green onion – spring onion – ayurved considers onion as rajasic and tamasic food. people who are engaged in pranayama – mediation avoid onion. It is sweet, little pungent, balances vata, neutral to pitta and increases kapha dosha.

Spring onions good for digestion can be used raw. During summer season people prefer to take it raw. it is used as a veggie, can be added in raita (kachumber).

All these leafy vegetables possess medicinal properties can be used by proper identification with local people of that particular area.

17. **Pudina** – Mint leaves – pungent, dry, light, balances kapha vata. it is used in many cuisines due to beautiful fragrance. It is an Aromatic herb used as carminative, digestive, appetizer, antispasmodic, antibacterial property. Pudina chutney is famous during rainy season specially used with pakora, bhujiya, samosa, chats, parathas. It stimulates stomach fire, though it is pungent it enhances taste. Pudina drink best remedy for stomach disturbances. Pudina is good kapha absorbent so used in kapha disorders. Pudina leaves boiled in water are good one to relieve gas (flatulence).

D. Fruits

fruits are good source to gain nutrients. we can use fruits any time anywhere, no need to process. Easy to digest, most people use fruits during fasting, as a substitute to meal. Many people use to maintain weight.

How to use fruits – common protocol

1. Use fresh seasonal fruits from local market.
2. Eat fruits which are available in your area.
3. Now a days Fruits are ripened artificially and made available for whole year. Avoid using frozen and preserved fruits.
4. Fruits can be consumed by grinding.
5. Some fruits can be used with cover as they are good for health and improves digestion like Chikoo, apple.
6. According to ayurved fruits must be taken with gap of 1- 2 hour from meal.

1. **Mango-** amra – mango is very important source of minerals and vitamins. it is favourite fruit of everyone. sweet mangoes are heavy, sweet, balances pitta vata and vitiates kapha dosha. Mangoes are available in variety dashara, kesar, hapus, kalmi, totapuri. Sour mangoes irritate pitta, kapha dosha and helps in digestion. Unripe mango is sour, astringent, pungent irritates pitta, vata and kapha also, improves tastes. Sweet mango helps in dhatuvruddhi, balkrut,shukrakar,nutritious, nourishing, improves sperm count,boosts strength.

   Sweet mango juice is preferred in Maharashtra with roti. Sweet mango juice is used with roti, puri, phulka, rice. Sour mangoes are used for variety of pickles, murramba, chutney, for sharbat. Amchur powder is used by drying the cover of raw mango which is used as flavour in sabji, dal. Mango seed has a medicinal property.

2. **Banana** – banana is widely available throughout the year. It is nutritious, delicious in taste. Good fruit for weight gaining. Ripened banana is heavy, sweet in taste balances vata, pitta. Ripe Bananas can be used as a breakfast menu or evening snack. Bananas are good source of minerals and vitamins. It is very easily available so easy to use. Banana smoothies are best nourishing drink. Bananas are good for school going children. raw bananas are sweet, astringent, heavy, cold vata pitta balancing, increases kapha dosha. Raw banana is used for making chips, sabji. banana stem, flower is used as food and medicine.

   Banana leaf is used from long as a traditional plate in many parts of India. people use banana leaf for pooja or rituals. Banana is widely used for various purposes for pooja, women offer as a custom during some festivals.

3. **Apple** – - seb - apple is most preferred fruit for patients. "An apple a day keeps doctor away "a famous quote. Apples are sweet heavy and cold in nature. Balances vata, pitta and increases kapha dosha.

Apples are rich source of fibres and minerals. Apples are good source of energy. Apples are eaten raw as a juice.

4. **Chikoo** – sapota – good source of calcium, iron. Light, cold and sweet in taste. Good for vata & pitta vitiates kapha dosha. Chikoo juice is good for nourishing dhatus.

5. **Guava** – amrud – Peru – guava is available in two variety white and pink. Rich source of fibre, mineral, vitamin C, astringent sweet in taste. Guava balances all three dosha. It improves digestion, good for stomatitis, improves liver function. It can be used raw, juice form, jam, chutney, sharbat, ice-cream.

6. **Jamun** – jambu – it is astringent, sweet, sour in taste. seasonal fruit available in rainy days. Balances kapha, pitta and irritates vata dosha. Fresh juice, powder is used as a medicine. If excess used causes constipation, it improves taste, anorexia.

7. **Grapes** – draksha - according to ayurved draksha is best fruit amongst all. Unripen grapes are sour in taste. Ripened grapes are sweet, unctuous, oily, heavy balances vata pitta. It helps for improving voice, soothing, good for respiratory system, gives strength, aphrodisiac in nature, cooling agent. dry grapes (raisins) are good for health, helps for smooth defecation, relives thirst, good source of minerals. 10 raisins soaked in water having good nutritional values during pregnancy, old age, children. raisins are used for garnishing the dishes. Grapes are contradicted with milk but raisins can be used in processed milk (masala milk).

8. **Pineapple** – ananas- Sweet, sour, heavy,balances vata pitta.

9. **Pomegranate** - dadim – anar – light, unctuous, sweet, sour in taste. Sweet pomegranate balances three dosha, sour increases pitta dosha. It is best used for thirst, burning sensation, boosts immunity, having aphrodisiac quality. In some parts of India, it is used with rice curd. It used for garnishing dishes, dabeli, fruit salad, raita, sharbat .

10. **Watermelon** - tarbuja – balances vata,kapha dosha increases pitta dosha. Juice of watermelon is best coolant drink.

11. **Custard apple** – Sitaphal -sweet in taste, cold potency, good for vata and pitta . Sitaphal vitiates kapha dosha. Good source for

magnesium, calcium and vitamins. Custard apples are good to increase strength.

12. Oranges – oranges are rich source of vitamin C . good for vata and kapha dosha. Sour, bitter and cold in potency. Orange juice is quick source of energy. Oranges boosts immunity. They drain up the excess mucus specially in respiratory system.

13. Papaya – papaya is good source of vitamin A and minerals. papaya is good for vata and kapha. It is perfect food or fruit for winter season as it gives heat. Ripened papaya is sweet in taste it helps to boost menstruation in females. It helps to improve digestion. If taken in excess quantity sometimes it upsets the stomach. Papaya leaves are good in fevers like dengue. Even papaya is good to overcome such type of diseases.

14. Fig – Anjeer - sweet and tasty fruit balances vata and pitta Dosha. Figs are good to balance thirst. overnight soaked dry figs helps in constipation as they are rich source of fibres and make stool soft. as they are naturally laxative can be used in diseases like piles, fissures or irritable bowel syndrome. Figs are good source of iron so beneficial in anaemia patients. In pregnancy they are good source of energy. Dried figs can be used by soaking overnight. Figs are rich source of calcium beneficial in osteoporosis and menopausal joint problems.

15. Cheri – cherries are good for mental and physical strength. Cherries are good source of vitamin C helps in boosting immunity. Cheri is included in diet plan as a salad and juice form. cherries are rich in antioxidant so good to consume for slowing the age.

E . Spices –

1. Cumin – jeerak - it is is the most useful spice used for making various dishes. light, dry, pungent in taste, balances kapha vata and irritates pitta dosha. Roasted Cumin powder is used as spice for making chutney, curry's, sambhar, pickles etc. cumin water is used during fever, cough, colic pain as a carminative, digestive drink.

2. Ginger – saunth, ardark is known to be vishwabheshaj in ayurved. Dry and fresh shunthi are having almost similar properties. Dry ginger is called as shunthi. Shunthi is Dry, pungent, heavy,hot in potency, balances kapha, due to pungent property irritates pitta dosha. Fresh ginger juice is good in kapha & vata vikar. For cough and cold ginger is used with gud and milk. It is best used as a digestive, carminative, appetizer. Shunthi tea is famous drink in winter. Shunthi water is best remedy for indigestion. Shunthi is used as a spice for making spicy sabji, non veg food, curries. small piece of ginger with black salt is a good appetizer.

3. Garlic – Rason – raw garlic sweet, salty, pungent, sour, bitter, astringent in nature. Garlic balances kapha vata and irritates pitta dosha. In India people use raw garlic for making Daal, sabji, chutney, pickles, masala powder.

4. Mirchi powder – red and green Mirchi are main variety of Mirchi used in kitchen. red Mirchi powder is pungent, hot in nature. green Mirchi is light, pungent. red Mirchi powder is widely used for taste and colour of food. It vitiates pitta dosha, balances kapha, vata. Excess use of Mirchi increases pitta leading ulcers, stomatitis, diarrhoea. Guntur, byadgi, Kashmiri Mirchi are some varieties of Mirchi. Mirchi is used to make food Spicer, it stimulates digestive juices. Green Mirchi is used for making chutney,thecha, paratha, puri, pakora etc. jowar roti and thecha is best menu for winter.

5. Green cardamon- Elechi - it is the cool spice used in Indian kitchen . it is pungent, dry, sweet, cold in potency, balances kapha & vata . it is used in masala tea, masala milk along with shunthi . it improves taste and flavour. It is used for garnishing sweets like semolina, kheer, porridges, shrikhand, barfi etc. it is useful in respiratory diseases like cough, cold, bronchitis. It helps to improve taste.

6. Turmeric – haldi – dry and wet turmeric both are used as food and medicine. Wet turmeric is used for making pickles, masala. Dry turmeric powder is used as colouring spice in Indian kitchen. Turmeric is best antimicrobial, antiviral, antibiotic. It is best for skin diseases, respiratory problems, diabetes, to improve immunity.

It can be used in food, along with milk, ghee, jaggery. It is bitter, pungent, dry in nature balances three dosha.

7. Clove – lavang, laung – bitter, pungent, oily balances pitta kapha dosha. Improves digestion, Appetizer, good for respiratory diseases, cough, cold, abdominal pain, asthma etc. clove oil is good for toothache, gargling in bad smell. Clove is used in tea masala, making black masala,

8. Marich -kali mirch, mire – it is pungent, hot in potency, balances kapha vata, increases pitta dosha. It used as spice for making sabji, soup, kadhi, masala buttermilk. it is used to improve taste as a carminative, Appetizer. Powder is used to treat cough cold. Mire powder is used along with honey, shunthi juice.

9. Mustard seeds – sarso, rai – it is used for giving tadka in Indian kitchen. Mustard seeds are available in variety, black, red, white, yellow black mustard are pungent increases pitta dosha. Red mustard is slightly sweet same as white mustard. Mustards are used for making sambhar masala, curries, daal, sabji,pickle. It used internally as well as externally. They are good carminative and digestives substance, improve taste.

10. Cinnamon – Twak – Dalchini – pungent, bitter, sweet, dry, light, increases pitta, balances vata kapha.

11. Fennel – Saunf - dry, sweet, pungent, astringent,bitter, balances vata kapha .fennel seed are tasty having specific flavonoids it can be used as a mouth freshener. Saunf is good for digestion, Saunf powder mixed with ajwayan, sugar, cinnamon is good for digestive health. Indian people use roasted fennel after meal for good digestion. Saunf water is good option for those suffering from indigestion, dyspepsia, anorexia.

12. Coriander seeds – dhania – astringent, bitter, hot in potency and balances three dosha. Coriander is a best friend of women, even many women don't cook food without coriander in kitchen. Green Coriander is used as spice, to improve taste and flavour of food for almost every dish. Green coriander almost available in every season. It is used as garnishing for poha, upma, sabji, chat items, chutneys, paratha, Daal, sambhar etc. kothimbir vadi is the famous one in Maharashtra . coriander seeds are cooling agent,

coriander drink is best for thirst, burning diseases, indigestion, acidity, dyspepsia, diarrhoea. Take 10 gm of coriander powder and add 10 parts of water to it keep for 8 – 10 hours, filter and use it. Sugar or jaggery can be added. It cleanses toxins like Ama, best for obesity, diabetes.

13. Ajayan – ajwain (Carom seeds)– ajwain seeds are best source of fibre, mineral. It is best digestive and carminative seed. Light, dry, pungent, bitter in taste. Ajwain balances kapha and vata vitiates pitta dosha. It is best anti-inflammatory, antibiotic. ajwain water is best for bloating, colic pain, indigestion, dyspepsia. It is safe to use in pregnant women.

F. Oils–

which oils are best for cooking commonly asked question but oils may be used according to requirement, many times it depends upon purpose like frying, cooking. oil make food edible, tasty, nourishing.

1. Sunflower oil – sunflower seeds are rich source of minerals. In India Oil is used for cooking. it balances vata pitta dosha.

2. Peanut oil – very commonly used oil for cooking specially in Maharashtra. peanuts are great source of protein, minerals. Peanuts are considered as legumes in ayurved. peanuts are used abundantly for making chutneys, laddu, chikki. peanut roti is famous dish during festive season in Maharashtra. Peanut oil is best for frying, cooking. It is good to lower bad cholesterol, cardiac health. Peanuts balances vata but irritates pitta, kapha dosha.

3. Sesame oil – sesame seeds are best nourishing seeds. sesame oil is used for cooking in some parts of India. Sesame seeds are hot, sweet, bitter in taste. sesame seeds are used as a great source of minerals for making chutney's, laddu, chikki . sesame oil is best for nourishing skin, hair, strengthen muscles. Sesame oil is best for vata, kapha, slightly increases pitta dosha.

4. Coconut oil – nariyal- coconut is cool, sweet nourishing in nature. coconut is used as a spice in Indian kitchen. Coconut is good for

weight gain, ojus building. Coconut oil is used for cooking, best for pitta, vata dosha. Coconut oil is used for dressing salads

5. Soyabean oil – soya is a good source of protein it is considered as a superfood now a days. Soyabean oil is used widely for cooking. It is good for metabolism specially omega – 3 fatty acids.

6. Cotton seed oil - in some parts of India cotton seed oil is used for cooking. It is good to increase good cholesterol and lower bad cholesterol.

7. Palm oil – palm oil contains saturated fats. daily use is not recommended, it is good to use for frying.

G. Nuts & Resins

1. almond – badam – vatad good for vata dosha, slightly increase pitta. Soaked almonds are good source of nutrition specially for vata dosha. Almonds are rich in protein, vitamin E, mg. almonds are used as whole as a energy boosting and weight gaining agent. almonds are used with milk for good health. Almonds are used as garnishing nut for sweet dishes like kheer, halva, laddu, barfi, cake, pastry etc to enhance taste. Ayurved recommend Almond with milk as lehya for children for weight gain, memory boosting, nerve tone.

2. cashews – cashews are sweet, cold balances vata, pitta and vitiates kapha dosha. Cashews are always taken with almonds in powder form with milk which boosts energy and fulfil daily requirement of nutrients. Cashews are used in curry's, pulao, sweet dishes.

3. raisins – dry grapes or raisins are used as a medicine for fever, burning diseases, thirst, mild laxative, vomiting. raisins are good source of fibres helps to boost energy, coolant to mind . balances vata, pitta and nourishes kapha. It is good to consume soaked raisins. raisins are used for garnishing food like halva, barfi, milk, kheer etc.

4. Pistachio – pista, yellow almond – good source of protein and phosphorous. It is used to garnish food.

5. Nutmeg – jaiphal – jaiphal is kitchen spice which is usually used for flavouring . it is added in very small amount to flavour the

food. nutmeg balances vata dosha. Nutmeg is used to relive stress and for sound sleep. Milk with little nutmeg powder is good to relive stress. Nutmeg also has some properties which helps for improving sexual life. It can be used as aphrodisiac drug.

6. Gond – gond is gum of tragacanth, edible gond can be taken from bark of tree. . it is of two types gond and gond katira . raw gond is good for health. gond is used for making laddu which is best during winter season to gain heat. Gond is dry, sticky low quantity is used. Gond can be taken by adding in milk or sweet menus. gond is a boon for pregnant and lactating women as it boosts lactation, helps for rejuvenation. Consume gond with milk those who are suffering from low back, joint pain, arthritis, neuropathies.

7. Dates – khajur – khajur is superfood used worldwide as a rich source of iron. Sweet, astringent, heavy cool in potency. khajoor is used during rituals like pooja, satynarayan. Khajoor is really nutritious, strengthens muscle, stimulates growth good source of energy for children, pregnant women, old age people. Khajoor is used for making laddu, chutney (sweet chutney for bhel – pani puri), kheer. khajoor water is good source of energy for burning diseases, haematuria, thirst, debility, blood diseases, diarrhoea etc. Soaked khajoor are good for constipation.

8. figs – anjeer – it is commercial fruit grown in various parts of India. Dry figs are good source of vitamins, minerals. calcium. it promotes growth, skin health, aging, wrinkles, good for stamina. Fig soaked in water are good to combat indigestion. In menopause or during pregnancy they really good source of calcium. Figs can be taken as food, dry anjeer, laddu, garnishing in sweets, anjeer jam, Murrumba .

9. Apricot – Jardalu – it is small yellow fruit; good source of iron can be used for vata balance.

10. Charoli – chironji – sweet, sour heavy to digest, balances vata pitta. improves skin tone, good for thirst, fever, burning sensation. chironji seed powder paste is used for skin problems like pimples, acne. Chironji seeds can be eaten raw also can be used with milk,

kheer, halva. chironji masala milk is preferred during Poornima to balance pitta dosha.

11. saffron – kesar – pungent, bitter, balances tridosha. Himachal region, Kashmir is the chief source of Saffron. saffron is the famous spice used due to its beautiful colour and fragrance. Kesar milk is highly recommended for pregnant women to improve baby's skin tone. kesar – badam milk is traditional recipe for improving vitality and to build ojus. It balances three dosha it is good to consume with milk for vata people. It is good to nourish dhatu and restore energy. Saffron is most precious as it is costly than other herbs.

12. sesame – sesame oil is great medicine which is widely preferred in ayurved. Sesame seeds are good source of protein and minerals. Black and white sesame seeds are little different in property. Sweet bitter in taste balances vata, kapha vitiates pitta dosha.

13. walnut – akrot – nutritious, oily, heavy to digest. walnuts balances kapha, vata and irritates pitta dosha. They are warm but astringent in nature so vata people should consume in powder form with milk or ghee. Walnut can be used by soaking for 5- 6 hours. Walnuts can be added in laddus.

14. Poppy seed – khas – khas – light, dry, bitter, astringent, balances vata and vitiates kapha dosha. Khas-khas is good nervous tonic as it lowers stress it enhances good and sound sleep. Khas – khas kheer is best remedy for insomnia. It is made by using coconut powder and milk. khas – khas kheer is given to puerperal women to strengthen nervous system and to balance vata dosha. Khas -kha seeds are widely used for garnishing cake, biscuits, cookies, pastries.

15. Pumpkin seed – sweet in taste in nature heavy to digest, irritates three dosha. Seeds are used for garnishing sweet food like kheer, barfi. pumpkin fruit is good for restoring health and used as a vegetable.

16. Arrroot – tavkheer – it is sweet in nature improves strength and vitality. It is consumed with milk for improving health.

17. Coconut – khobra - coconut is heavy, oily, sweet, cold in nature it is good for vata, pitta . it is good for weight gain, strength. Dry

coconut is used as a spice in Indian kitchen for making curries, non-vegetarian food items, chutney, laddu. coconut milk is used for laddu, kadhi. Coconut water is coolent and rich in mineral used to sustain energy in diarrhoea, dysentery, dehydration. Coconut pulp is used for nourishment.

18. Peanut – moong Fali - peanuts are described as legumes in ayurved. Peanuts are rich in vitamin and minerals. Peanuts are used as raw and as oil. Peanuts are largely used raw as snack. Roasted peanuts with salt, boiled peanuts with salts are consumed as evening snack. Peanuts balances vata dosha, vitiates pitta and kapha. Roasted Peanut powder is used for making vegetables. Peanuts are used for chutney, laddu, chhikki which is nutritious and good to increase haemoglobin.

H. **Dairy Products**

1. Milk –

    Milk – Dudh . 8 types of milk are described in ayurved. Milk is nutritious, rich source of calcium, protein. Milk is first food for child. Daily Milk consumption is recommended as a medicine in many diseases like peptic ulcer (grahni), rajyakshma (tuberculosis), debility, anaemia. Cows milk is sattvik and good among all milk. Researches shown that cows milk is good source of energy, ojus, improves vitality, balances vata pitta.

    Milk is used for various purposed making medicine, for Basti (enema), shirodhara (pouring on head), Gandush (gargling).

    Mothers milk (stree Dugdh) – ayurved highly recommends mothers milk for neonates as it is light, easily digestible, vital, good for health. It can be used for Nasya and Aschyotan procedure.

How to consume milk – general guidelines for

a. According to Ayurved milk can be taken separately as a breakfast in morning which is beneficial to strengthen the body.

b. can add sugar, jaggery, masala to improve taste.

c. vata – pitta people - warm milk can be taken in morning after breakfast. For vata it is better to take milk with fat as they need nourishment.

d. kapha people can take milk (low fat or without fat) but with using spices like green cardamom, turmeric, kesar . you can add water to make it low fat.

e. milk can be consumed at night at least 1 hour before bed for good sound sleep and as a nutrient for elders, children's, pregnant women.

f. milk can be taken with nut powder, dates in general debility, children's, pregnancy, puerperal stage.

g. ayurved recommends raw milk (not processed such as pasteurization), it is better to take milk from village sources (milk man). Raw milk is boiled for at least 5 minutes then it can be used.

2. Butter - - makkhan – Navneet – butter is sweet in taste, balances vata pitta and vitiates kapha dosha. Butter is favourite one of lord krishna. Butter is used with roti, pulao, paratha. Bajara roti with makkhan is good one during winter season. Butter is good aphrodisiac, rich source of vitamin D, A, K, E .

3. Buttermilk – Mattha – Takra – ayurved recommend Takra as nectar on earth. Takra can be made by adding adequate quantity of water in curd (2 part = 2 part) . churning action make this very light so it is better to consume buttermilk rather than curd. Butter milk is light to digest, carminative, Indian people are big fan of mattha (masala buttermilk) which is prepared specially by adding spices like cumin, dhania, ajwain powder to the buttermilk. Sweet lassi made by adding sugar and green cardamom. Buttermilk is super medicine for indigestion, irritable bowel syndrome,

haemorrhoids, ascites. buttermilk is good to pacify vata dosha, it vitiates pitta and kapha. Pitta can take by adding sugar, kapha by adding salt. As it is hot not recommended in hot weather. In Gujrat, Panjab, Maharashtra people daily consume buttermilk with salt.

4. Ghee – ghrit, sarpi – ghee is very beneficial and important part of diet. Ghee is good for vata pitta and it vitiates kapha dosha. Ghee is sweet, cold, stimulates digestive fire, memory, good for complexion, increases immunity, vital to life. ghee balances vata pitta, kapha can use little amount. Cows' ghee is cold in potency balances vata pitta, gives strength to mind and body.

    Ghee is auspicious as it is used for ancient periods for pooja (ghee ka Diya), special occasions like Navratri, Shravan month ghee lamping is good for positive vibrations and energy. Ghee – roti, ghee – rice is very good appetizer recommended for children's, old age persons. ghee is used in Indian kitchen for making laddu, halva, sweets, barfi etc. it is best used with roti, daal, rice, milk. In Indian custom ghee is served with food as ghee is sattvik it creates positiveness and increases the vitality of food. Milk and ghee are good combination for strength and rejuvenation, relives constipation. Ayurved recommends old ghee as it much beneficial. for sound sleep ghee with milk is good before one hour of going bed. for memory and concentration ghee and milk can be used in day time also. Fatty people, during cough and cold ghee is not recommended. Ghee can be used with warm water if milk is not preferable. Ghee is good aphrodisiac can be used in infertility, low sperm count, debility etc. vata people can use 2- 3 tsp. ghee, pitta can use 1-2 tsp. and kapha may use occasional (weekly 3 times – 1-2 tsp.).

5. Milk skin – milk skin is good for rejuvenation, strength. Milk skin is utilised for making ghee. It can be taken with roti, rice.

6. Paneer – panner is proceed from curdling of milk. Now a days people are using it for protein supplement. It is good source of protein calcium. Paneer is used for making pakora, sabji, paratha

etc. according to ayurved vata people can use paneer, pitta can use moderately, kapha person very occasionally as it irritates kapha .

7. Cheese – cheese is made by curdling of protein in milk. Cheese balances vata dosha, not good for kapha dosha, neutral to pitta. Sweet and heavy to digest. Not indicated during kapha time.

8. Khava – khoya – full of fat, sweet, balances vata, pitta and increases kapha dosha. Khoya is good source of vitamin B12 - riboflavin, vitamin D . khoya having same benefits like that of milk. khoya is used for making sweets, roti, halva, Gulab jamun etc. khoya is good for strengthening bone, weight gain,

9. Curd – according to ayurved curd is hot, improves digestive power, heavy to digest, increases kapha pitta, balances vata dosha. Fresh curd is good probiotic. ayurved recommends curd should be taken with Amalki, jaggery, green gram, honey. Curd can be used with roti, paratha, puri, rice etc. in India daily fresh curd is prepared and utilised. curd is good if taken with sugar and jaggery. Curd is not recommended at night unless it is consumed with sugar, green gram or jaggery, As it is kapha time curd increases kapha dosha. Pitta people should consume little curd with sugar. At ancient times curd was prepared in clay pot (matka) . curd is not recommended in inflammatory diseases, skin diseases.

I Bakery products – ayurved don't recommend bakery products much as they are made by fermentation process and becomes heavy to digest probably routine use causes low stomach fire. Most of bakery products are made by using items like Maida, grains (corn, wheat) yeast and oil. Bakery products are easy to carry, serve, good source of energy, fibres but difficult to digest according Indian weather conditions. As they lower the digestive power so not to consume much.

1. Bread – bread is flat dove made by process of fermentation of yeast, grains. If bread is made by using nutritious grains like, wheat, corn, millets. breads are great source of fibres, vitamin b complex like thiamine, niacin. Bread is used as main meal in all countries. In India bread is used in breakfast or making menus like pizza, chivda etc. bread can be made without yeast with whole grains

and water. You can add some spices like green cardamom, kesar for flavour. Bread and tea or milk may be preferable for vata and pitta people.

2. Pav – pav is another form of bread having same properties like bread. Pav is quite popular in India as ladi pav – (as this is made by using pav- feet). Pav is served with famous dish pav- bhaji. Pav can be use with milk or tea. Vada- pav, missal - pav, Dabeli, pav – chutney is some famous dish. pav is made by using Maida and all-purpose flour. Pav is not mush good according to ayurved as it is heavy to digest, pav is soft then bread. Good source of carbohydrates so vata pitta can use in little, kapha should avoid.

3. Cakes – cakes are made up of Maida, white sugar, ghee, oil salt, butter. cake is good for vata, pitta but vitiates kapha dosha. Cakes are not recommended for kapha vitiated diseases like diabetes, obesity, skin allergies etc. we can use flours like wheat, corn, oat, almond and coconut. instead of artificial sweeteners we can go with honey, jaggery, banana, apple, dates. according to dosha we can add spices, for vata ginger, piplai, for pitta – green cardamom, for kapha ginger, clove, cardamom. In such a way we can make some changes.

4. Cream rolls – cream rolls are made by Maida, oil, sugar, cream. They are rich in protein and fat. Vata, pitta can use moderately, kapha should avoid.

5. Biscuits – cookies - biscuits are made by using grains like wheat, millet, corn, oat etc. biscuits are very preferable and favourite menu for each one. biscuits are very easy to use any time anywhere. many people use tea / milk – biscuits in breakfast. biscuits are good for vata and pitta, vitiates kapha dosha. Not recommended in kapha diseases like diabetes, obesity, low stomach fire, indigestion. Now a days special ayurvedic biscuits are available for each dosha type. For vata, we can add cardamom, kesar, nuts, ghee, dates, coconut. For pitta we can add coconut, gulkand, Indian gooseberry, for kapha ajwain, Pippali, turmeric, cumin etc. we can fruit pulp, watermelon seeds, spices, green gram, rice flour according to dosha . shatavari, ashwangdha Pippali, musali biscuits are available in market. Khari and sweet bicuits are

6. Toast – toast is type of bread which is made by browning with heat. simply in kitchen when we roast bread in iron pan it becomes pink red it is said to be toast. Toast can be eaten with tea or masala milk. We can add spices like cumin, ajwain, toast are good in carbohydrates and low in protein, fat. We can use toast by adding toppings like butter, vegetables, jams, sauces etc.

7. Khari – khari is another version of toast which is made by adding abundant amount of ghee, butter or vanaspati oil. It can be flavoured by spices like cumin, ajwain, Hing. khari can be eaten with tea and milk. Kharis are more crispy and crunchy. vata, pitta people can use, kapha should avoid it.

8. Donuts - donuts are smooth,flavoury and tastes good. Donuts are made of wheat flour, Maida, sugar, salt, butter, milk, yeast . donuts are good for vata and pitta, irritates kapha dosha. Moderate use is good, regular use increase weight and load on heart.

9. puffs – puffs are available in variety like veg & non veg. puff is combination of vegetables and flour. They are made by using flour, steamed vegetables, spices, butter, salt etc. puffs are favourite evening snack preferred in town and metro cities.

10. Pastry – pastry another form of cakes. pastries are preferred by children. pastries are not good for kapha dosha, vata, pitta can use moderately. Process of making pastries is same with cakes. Baking, decoration ideas, colours are utilized differently.

11. Muffins – muffins are spongy like cakes, small in size, less sugary.

12. Cadbury / chocolate – Cadbury or chocolate are favourite one for each one. Chocolate is sign of love and attachment. ayurveda says that as it is made of coco powder which is bitter, light and cold it is not good for vata dosha. Pitta can use moderately, for kapha bitter taste is ok but as it is sweet avoid overuse. People use chocolate as a mood elevator as it stimulates serotonin

Chapter 8

Utensil for cooking

If we see the Vedic culture of cooking clay pots (mitti Ka Ghada – Matka) are used to make food. In the ancient period food is directly kept on fire as no utensils are available and served on leaves. as per revolution slowly clay pots are being used for cooking purpose. Afterwards metals like brass, silver, copper, iron are being popular during mid period. Silver, gold plates, cups, jars are popularly used by kings and landholders or by rich people.

During the period of roman (8th century) most of the utensils are discovered.

Afterwards steel, aluminium become popular among common people. Aluminium pans are still used for cooking food. Steel plates, jars, glass and other variety is used in Indian kitchen for serving, storing food. In 1950 around copper glass or jars preferred for storing water due to its health benefits. In 20th century steel for serving, storing, aluminium, copper bottom pans are being used for cooking food. In 21st century non- stick pan become popular as they are easy to handle. Now we are using variety of metals for various purposes . steel for storing, serving, copper for drinking water, aluminium -cooking, chinimati – cups saucers. Glass is being used from olden times specially to serve the liquids and to store the pickles or some special food. From last decade plastic is very much popular in metro cities for storing and serving food due to its easy handling. but now it is banned as many diseases like cancer, skin allergies to be due to overuse of plastic

Type of utensil	Uses – benefits	Dosha prefers	Special indications
Clay	For cooking, storing water, buttermilk, curd	Good for all type of dosha person	Curd, buttermilk tastes good
Brass	Storing, cooking,	Moderate use for all types	Cooked food should be removed immediately in another pan
Iron	For cooking	Good for all dosha as iron is good for blood formation	Cooked food should be removed immediately in another pan to avoid complications
Gold	Cooking, serving	It is auspicious for all dosha	On special occasion golden utensils are preferred which balances three dosha
Silver	Serving, storing	Good for pitta, vata	Good for immunity energy, milk is served in silver pot (aphrodisiac)
Steel	Cooking, serving, storing	Can be used by all	Tea, milk well stored in steel pot
Melanin	Serving	Better to avoid for all	
Stones – soapstone vessels	Khalva – churning chopping vessels are made by stone. traditionally pots are used for grinding, cleaning grains.	Sambar, rasam, curry's, buttermilk is well cooked in stone vessels . it is healthy to cook in stone vessels.	
Wood	Wooden pots are used to store food specially rotis, bread	It is good for health. as it keeps roti, chapati in good condition	Rural people use wooden pot (circular) specially to store roti, chapati. now many uses hot pot to store roti.

China clay – bone China – porcelain	Widely used for making tea cups, crockery's	Used widely for storing serving food	Can sustain heat. traditionally pickles are best stored in porcelain pots for a long.
Cast iron	Cooking specially roasting – tava pan	It is good for all dosha	Cast iron is popular in kitchen as it can be used for high temperatures
Aluminium	Cooking, storing	Used widely for cooking food	Sour food, curd, kadhi, buttermilk is not served or stored in aluminium utensils
Metal	Better to avoid cooking in metals but if used remove immediately in another pan.	Not good for all type	Can be used for storage of grains
Branz (kansa)	Cooking, serving	Vata pitta	Kapha. ayurved recommends cooking is good in branz vessels
Non stick	Cooking, storing	Used widely for making food but researches shows that not beneficial for health	The coating of metal is not good for health
Glass -	Serving, storing	Balances all dosha, beverages like juice, sharbat, water, buttermilk, wine is served in glassware's	Glass is transparent metal so widely used for beverages as it looks beautiful with different variety and colours.
Plastic	Serving, storing	Ayurved not recommend use of plastic	Not beneficial for health

Leaves – banana, swede, neep, snagger, turnip, rutabaga, banyan, Sal tree, Kamal, cinnamon, turmeric, Ficus leaves are used for making plates.	Used to cover food for some special dishes, serving in banana leaf is auspicious. all these leaves are used to make plate,	Balances all three dosha. ayurved recommends leaf's for lepa and covering wound	It is custom to use banana leaves during rituals like marriage, pooja. many leaves are used to offer navaidyam, prasad after pooja .Tamilnādu, Karnataka, kerla, Andhra Pradesh, kokan, goa uses plates and bowls for serving food .

Storage of food

Classically food can be stored in following ways.

Water	Copper enhances the qualities beneficial for balancing dosha
Milk	Steel, glass, silver
Drinks – juices or any liquid	Better to store in silver
Fruits, vegetables, snacks	Pot made by leaves as it keeps fruits fresh
Cooked meat	Silver is better but can be stored in glass, China, stell pots
Pickles	Porcelain pots
Sour, cooked buttermilk	Stone vessels
Wine, syrups	Glass vessel
Ghee	Glass container

Chapter 9

Food for specific age group

Ayurvedic classics explains how to feed neonates uniquely. Kashyap Samhita is one of the oldest classics which gave detail explanation of diet.

Ayurved categorizes age in three

Avastha	Years	Dosha dominance	Key points
1. Balyavastha (childhood) –	1- 16 yrs.	Kapha dominance	Growth, nourishment,
2. Madhyam – middle age	16 – 60 yrs.	Pitta dominance	Power, vitality, completeness, decision making
3. Vardhakya – geriatric age –	Above 60 yrs.	Vata dominance	Debility, degenerative changes

A. Balayavstha - childhood

1. Kshirad (only milk) upto six months
2. kshirannad (milk and food) – six months to one and half years
3. Annadad (food) – from two years

1. **kshirad** –
   a. **First four months** – only milk after birth within 4- 5 hours first feed should be given to neonate, if mother is settled

down. mothers' milk has lots of good properties which are beneficial for growth, development, immunity of neonate. Ayurved highly recommends mothers milk as it is superfood for child. In absence of mother another woman (close relative) can also feed baby. Ayurved recommends lehan (gold, nuts are used for same purpose) . this is given early morning empty stomach which is good option for immunity.

b. **four to six months** – milk and other liquids like – soup, fruit juice, tomato juice, vegetable soup, orange juice as per the availability and choice.

c. **Six months –** at the age of sixth months baby can take juicy semisolid food material which is easy to swallow.

We can give carbohydrate and protein substances which helps for growth. We may give vegetable soup, soft rice, moong Daal khichari, nachani with milk, Satu with milk or water.

1. Khichari recipe- rice and moong (splinted) - 2 cups – roast this and make a fine powder in mixi . now take 1 cup water boil add one spoon powder to it cook, add little ghee or milk and salt for taste. Make thick as baby can easily consume. this is superfood for baby.
2. Nachani – 1 spoon Nachani powder can be used by cooking in milk or water.
3. Satu - 1 spoon powder can be used by cooking in milk or water.
4. Vegetables – thin soup is made by boiling vegetables like cabbage, spinach, tomatoes, corn etc.
5. Semolina – sweet or spicy semolina can be given.
6. Porridges – made by wheat and milk is healthy
7. Mix cereals – take wheat, jowar, Nachani, moong, Toor roast and make fine powder, it can be used by cooking in milk and water .

8. Fruit juices – mango, apple, oranges, papaya – cooked preferred. Juices can be given. Bananas are good as sweet taste baby easily prefers.
9. Nuts powder – almond, cashews, raisins, dry dates powder is used with milk.
10. Egg white portion – if preferred can give nonveg soups also.

2. **Kshirannada - Six months to one and half years** – above same can be used as baby's teeth grows you can use solid food slowly. Sweet taste is preferred as it helps growth and nourishment.
3. **Annada** – 2 years above – Now child can take solid foods as a part of regular diet. as per growth and nutrition is considered it is better to give, sweet, soft, simple, nutritious homemade food including proteins, carbohydrates, fats and vitamins, sattvic food.

Important components – cereals, milk, curd, buttermilk, leafy vegetables, seasonal fruits, ghee, jaggery eggs, nuts.

We must teach children good food habits, include variety of food. avoid chocolates, cold drinks, processed food, instant food, tea coffee.

a. Healthy tiffin menus – vegetable paratha, roti – sabji, Daal rice, sweet roti, occasionally puri, porridges, salads, laddus, nuts, chikkis, fruit chat etc.

b. Dosha food -

This is kapha phase of life so kapha disorders are more likely to be occur. Use spices adequately to make up with kapha dosha.

If child is overactive, irritative in nature, less memory, underweight (vata character) use food wisely which is nutritious, sattvik food like milk, butter, makkhan, ghee, jaggery, dates, bananas, fresh food preferred. Avoid dry frozen food.

If child is hyperactive, stubborn, ambitious, arrogant use food which is cooling, calming like kheer. Halva, milk, ghee, fresh food.

c. **food during puberty** – drastic changes in personality are seen during puberty stage. At the age of 8- 9 years puberty changes are seen in girls. at the age of 11-12 most of the girs are menstruating needs special care. As girls enter in puberty they start thinking about figure and beauty avoid certain nutritious things, and prefer processed packed foods. Mother should strictly advise to take balances homemade diet. fiberize, roughages, milk, vegetables, soyabean products, carrots, banana, apple, cereals in diet.

4 to 5 meals are preferred.

B. Madhyam vaya - Middle age 16 to 60

This is golden period of everyone's life. One can do whatever he wants. in this stage of life diet depends upon pattern of work, requirements according to time (age). Balanced three to four meals are required. Adequate number of fibres, vitamins (A, K, C), minerals are needed.

One can take food according to constitution (details are given in chapter).

This period we can divide as upto forty and afterwards. Upto forty-one can eat and digest well afterwards digestive power reduces slowly.

Common tips for planning meal

1. Plan meal as per your Agni (stomach fire).
2. if we consume only carbohydrates they are digested soon, if we consume only fat or only protein it will take time for digestion, so diet should be balanced with all three. Each meal should be balanced.
3. don't include so many food items in one meal.
4. don't combine many fatty foods in one meal
5. prepare food in variety with colour, odour and taste.

C. **vardhakya – old age** – old age is again considered as balyavstha (childhood). Lowered dhatu bala, lowered stomach fire, dryness, fatigue, low immunity are some common signs of old age. key factors of diet are soft, warm, nutritive, nourishing, soothing. One should include simple, homemade food which can be easily digested. Roti, vegetables, Daal, rice, fruits, nuts can be included in diet.

Breakfast – milk, porridges, daal -rice, semolina, paratha,
Lunch -roti sabji, dal, rice, buttermilk, salad
Evening snack – laddu, masala milk, any seasonal fruit,
Dinner – khichari, soup, curry's, pulao
Occasional – as per preferences sweet, spicy food can be taken.

General tips

1. Plan meal as per your intake capacity.
2. See for any specific age-related health problems like hypertension, diabetes, cardiac issues.
3. Make sure that diet should be healthy and nourishing.
4. Include milk, ghee, buttermilk adequately .
5. Soaked almonds, raisins helps for easy defaecation.
6. Avoid overeating or dieting.
7. Dates, sesame, coconut, bananas, tofu, are beneficial'
8. Stay away from stale, processed refined food, cold drinks, frozen food.
9. Don't eat in noisy environment or weather.
10. Eat in relaxed mood, don't eat in stressed mood.
11. Eat on regular time, make a timetable or food chart and display it near the dining room that keep you updated.
12. Focus on health issues.
13. Prefer cooked food rather than raw.
14. Ojus and

E . Diet during pregnancy

Pregnancy (garbhavastha) is precious period of life. Ayurveda has a great contribution in planning meal during nine months of period. Monthly regimen is indicated according to growth and development of foetus.

Month	Diet
Month one	Sweet cold and liquid, congenial diet (satmya bhojan) 2-3 times a day. (If patient is suffering from hyperemesis warm, soft, less spicy, dry food) masala milk (cardamom, kesar, turmeric) or plain milk with sugar. Include ghee, halva, porridges in diet.
Month two	Milk process with herbs like shatavari, Ashwagandha. Sweet, cold, liquid diet. add seasonal fruit, nuts as per preferences
Month three	Milk, honey and ghee, khichari (moong and rice), rice and milk, sweet taste is preferred all over pregnancy .
Month four	Butter with milk, milk and cooked rice, it's good to take food which is pleasant to that women . warm, fresh homemade food is preferred. Curd rice is good option.
Month five	Ghee and milk, rice with milk, meat (if preferred), rice gruel cooked in milk, sweet kheer of rice (can add cold spices like cardamom, coconut, nuts)
Month six	Ghee, ghee with rice or roti, sweet curd
Month seven	Ghee, milk, sweets made up of milk or ghee
Month eight	Gruel cooked with milk and ghee, liquid items, soft food, meat soup, sweets made by milk and ghee
Month nine	Meat soup, rice gruels, cereals, milk

Overall sweet, nourishing, refreshing food is preferred throughout pregnancy. Better to avoid sharp, hot, spicy, stale, fermented, processed food.

During first three months women suffers from anorexia, loss of appetite to pacify pitta dosha (acidity) sweet food is preferred. Milk and ghee pacify pitta and improves Agni. milk completes nutritional requirements and balances fluid level.

After first trimester major changes are observed in foetus. Next trimester (4 to 6 month) is of Growth and nourishment. meat soup, butter provides best nourishment.

In later trimester due to weight gain most of the women may have oedema on feet, face. diuretic herbs are beneficial for such condition. In last month many women may suffer constipation to avoid it milk, ghrit are beneficial.

Along with all this one should follow seasonal regimen also.

Preferred Food list

1. Moong	11. Pomegranate
2. Wheat	12. Banana
3. Toor	13. Kesar
4. Shashtik shali	14. Dates
5. Laja	15. Grapes
6. Jaggery	16. Mango
7. Milk	17. Makkhan
8. Honey	18. Amla
9. Ghee	19. Sugar
10. Buttermilk	20. Meat soup
	21. Curd

A. Diet During Menopause

Menopause is cessation or stoppage of bleeding (can happen in age 40 to 50 yrs.) Some common symptoms of menopause are dryness, mood swings, hot flashes, irregular menses, weight gain, sleep disturbances and many more. Menopause is transitional natural phase of life many women can easily accept, but for many it is troublesome.

More carbohydrates, fat & proteins moderately, minerals in good quantity is basic need during menopause.

As it is vata phase one should avoid vata diet. Plan diet as per your dosha and symptoms of menopause.

Menopause type	Food preferences	Avoid food
1. Vataj – dryness, fatigue, bone problems, joint pain, sleep disturbances, disturbances in digestion	Moist, warm, fresh, nutritious, nourishing Breakfast – milk (masala), oats, sweet items, Lunch – regular congenial meal with ghee, sweets Dinner – before 7.00 pm Take milk – at night for good sound sleep Use spices like cumin, turmeric, ginger, ajwain, Soaked raisins, almonds good for nourishment. Chavanprash, shatavari powder with milk is good to maintain strength .	Dry, frozen, stale, carbonated beverages
Pittaj menopause	Moist, cool, sweet, bitter taste is preferred. Use cool spices like dhaniya, cumin Breakfast – nourishing, cool Lunch – simple, homemade, less spicy, Dinner- rice daal, ghee Use milk, ghee, buttermilk, amala, gulkand	Spicy, hot, pungent, salty, sour, processed, instant, pickles, chats
Kaphaj menopause	Dry, warm, bitter. roasted, use less oil and water for making food. Breakfast – warm water, kadha, soup Lunch – less oily steamed food, use spices, phulka Dinner- khichari, soup	Sweet, salty, sour, moist, fatty,

Along with diet one can follow healthy lifestyle, pranayama, yoga, concentration practices for happy menopause.

Chapter 10

Disease wise Diet

1. Vataj vyadhi

<ul><li>Vata dosh is dry, rough, cool, light and mobile in nature. One should consume food which work on these properties . opposite food like oily, warm, moist, heavy, nourishing is useful to balance the vata dosha.</li><li>Wheat roti, kheer, shashtisali rice – cooked well with ghrut is best for vata.</li><li>Any sweet dish like sweet semolina, laddu, chikkis, biscuits, khajur, jaggery, honey are good to use.</li><li>Lady's finger, dudhi, brinjal can be used.</li><li>moong, black gram, horse gram, Toor can</li><li>be used by cooking well with masalas.</li><li>Fruits like pomegranate, mangoes, tamarind, lemon, grapes are used.</li><li>Ginger, curcumin, onion, carrot, radish can be used by various dishes like halva, pickles, veggies.</li><li>Tambula, mishri, castor oil, Madya, musta water, coconut water, sarshap, Haleem</li></ul>	

b. Gout (vatarakta) use Old rice, Shastisali rice, wheat . Use guduchi veggi, spinach, tandulja,karela Use moong soup, massor, toor,vatana . Kapoor water, dhania- cumin water, lajamand, Use lajamand add khandsharkara, Kapoor and use it reduces kleda. Harataki churn, old jaggery, katha mix and use.	
c. Rheumatoid Arthritis – (Amavata) - Old cereals specially varai, Nachani, Satu . Karela, shigru, spinach can be used frequently. Kulthi, Toor masoor used as sprouts. Use ginger, garlic, carrot, onion, turmeric. Use castor oil, gomutra, bhallatak, ajwayan,saunth, saunuf, Hing. Use castor oil 1- 6 tsp. at night every month to relief from constipation. 1tsp. Garlic juice, 1 tsp. saunth, castor oil relieves pain. Satu flour, rice flour, add castor oil and make roti. Use garlic coriander chutney, kulthi pithle (sabji),karela sabji. For acidity use wet turmeric pickle. Karela chutney, Padwal subji. Use kulthi (hoarse gram) and chana soup add Hing, mire, saindhav, sunthi, garlic in it. Use warm water, non-veg people can use goat meat .	

C. Abdomen pain (Udershool) v eat Ginger piece with saindhav before meal, can add Hing, ajwayan, black salt,ghrut, makkhan for vatanuloman. Moong soup, sharbat (mango, mint, ajwayan, orange, nimbu, saunf pineapple with black salt)Ajwayan, cumin, souf, sunthi, balantshepa(shatpushpa) equal amount roast it and add saindhav, black salt, Hing in it. Take this 4 times in a day drink warm water. 1 tsp. Ghrita half tsp. ajwayan, l garlic kali eat this with first bite, use ghrita in meal. Take shrabat by using warm water, grape, amla, nimbu. Drink castor oil for doshprashman. dadim juice, coconut water, nimbu sharbat. Rice kheer, phulka with ghrit, brinjal veggi, Padwal, chakwat, karela chutney, Khobar chutney, kokam pickle, amla pickle, makkhan	
D. Arochak (anorexia) - Ghrut, buttermilk, curd, milk, shrikhand, • Musta jal, saunth jal, Ushnodaka, • Garlic, ginger, moola, carrot, onion • Black sesame, black salt – gargling • Kankol churn, supari – mukhshudhdi • Amla, dalchini • Food with low calorie and low fat is good to use. • More proteins are useful to stay longer. • Warm water is beneficial, avoid cold water. • Use lemon juice in food items.	

• Avoid fried items instead use boiled / steamed food or vegetables. • Small divided meals are better to use to lower food cravings. • Low fat milk is preferred. • Include food like amla (Indian gooseberry), karela (bitter gourd), madhu (honey), moong (green gram),yava (barley), anar (pomegranate), mattha (masala buttermilk). • Use cabbage s much as possible.	
E.Kashtartav – (dysmenorrhea) Consume ginger tea is beneficial, you can add basil leaves or jaggery in it. Take cumin water – boil two glass water with 1 tsp. cumin, make it half and use. You can add honey or jaggery in it. Use ajawain water, or saunf water t relieve pain. Garlic clove and cloves paste is useful – you can add in water or as a powder form. Nimbu sharbat, raw mango sharbat are also effective . Drink warm water as much as possible to stay hydrated. Take Tub bath or steam to lower abdomen. Cooling bath is also effective to relieve stress. Add spices like lahsun, cumin, Hing, mint, coriander in preparing food. Bananas, pomegranate, raisins, grapes are beneficial .	

F.(Amenorrhoea) – Anartav- Use of properly prepared decoction of Krishna Tila mixed with Jaggery in the morning, induces menstruation in a woman having amenorrhea for a very long time. • Use of decoction of Manjishtha and Lavang . Lashuna should be included in diet, diet made with barley, milk, Mamsarasa, Sidhu, powdered Pippali & Bala Tail are beneficial in Yonirogas.	

G. rajaksheenta (scanty menses) Til gud kwath
 	
   • Phulka – Methi, shigru, chutney (sesame, karela, garlic), kulthi(horse gram) curry, metkut (mix daal chutney),buttermilk after lunch
   • Methi powder, jaggery, ghee – laddu
   • Haleem kheer
   • Buttermilk with masala – mattha
   • Kulthi kwath
   • Papaya
   • Cumin fant + souf
   • Kharwas
   • Mangoes, amra Paak, coconut barfi, kohla (petha), eggs, milk, honey
   • Beet, moola, cabbage,kachumber can be taken.
   • Spinach soup – garlic, onion, Hing, cumin	

H. Shwetpradar – (leucorrhea) Banana + Ela, banana + makkhan, banana+ mishri
 	
   • Amla churna honey
   • Rice with milk + ghee (rice without salt, you can make gruel)	

• Gulkand, milk • Tandulja juice • Rice water (tandulodak) • Coconut barfi, kohla barfi • Fenugreek water • lady's finger – boil – make paste • Spinach, broccoli, garlic, nuts, flex seeds • Tulsi kwath with honey • Pomegranate • Banana flower juice is used by mixing with honey and sugar. • Banana with mishri or makhan is also good remedy. • Rice water along with cumin powder and jaggery is quick beneficial remedy. • Cooked rice can be eaten by adding jaggery and cumin. • Buttermilk with amla powder is good one to relieve from leucorrhoea.	
I. Raktapradar – Dysfunctional Uterine bleeding • Roti – phulka, banana (kelphul sabji), amla pickle, moong daal, soft rice ghee, • Dadim juice, banana with green cardamom, • Wheat porridge – phulka, corn starch (Araroot), singhada kheer • Mamsarasa siddh rice with ghee • goat Soup • Gond laddu, Haleem kheer, khajur, singhada laddu • Half supari, 1 tsp. Amla churn – 2,3 times a day	

J. Madhumeha –(Diabetes) Anna varg – wheat old, Satu,varai, nachani, jowar (yellow).
 	
  • Shaak – shigru, methi, karela, Padwal, kamalkand
  • Shimbi varg – kulthi, Toor, chana, masoor, moong, mataki
  • Fruits – umber, raw banana, jambu, kapith, khajur,
  • Buttermilk, warm water, shrutsheet Jala, garlic,ginger, turmeric, carrot, onion,
  • Sesame, clove, Ela, khaskhas, tamalpatra
  • For frequency of urine- Bilva swaras 2-2 tsp. turmeric juice
  • Banana flower sabji, sesame, jowar roti, karela, cabbage, kulthi pithle
  • Jambu beej churn with buttermilk, ajwayan powder,
  • Methi laddu
  • Ginger juice – garlic
  • Laja -	

K. Fever – jware Fasting, For thirst laja water can be used. Amla water, sugarcane juice, grape juice, Dadim juice, musta water, ushnodak, ginger tea, shabudana kanji, dhaniya water, moong soup	

L. Pandu – (anaemia)

cereals – wheat, jav, jowar, moong, masoor, Toor

- Vegetables – cabbage, Padwal, brinjal, tandulja, shepu
- Fruits – amla, Draksh, Anjir, oranges, chiku, Dadim, banana, mango, apple
- Panchagavya all
- Ginger, turmeric, garlic, onion, radish, sesame oil, keshar, khajur, Nagkeshar
- Shinghada flour with, roasted khajur eat early morning. After one hour drink cow's milk.
- Black raisin water, sugarcane juice, bhumiamla juice, amla juice
- Palpitation – louki juice cumin powder
- For constipation amla munnka water is best.
- Chincha panak
- Kanji, buttermilk,
- Drink amla juice and red beetroot help reactivate red blood cells
- soak 2-3 tsps. of fenugreek (Methi) seeds overnight. Add these seeds to rice and cook them. Put salt as required, you can eat Methi rice.
- mix half a cup of apple juice with half a cup of beetroot (chaukidar) juice and take for month.
- Soak black sesame (til) seeds in warm water for at least 2 hours. Make the paste of it and add honey to the mixture. Then, mix well, put in the glass of milk, and have it daily.
- Eat a pomegranate (Anar) to increase your blood count.

• bananas to increase the hemoglobin count. • Eat green leafy vegetables like spinach, peas, beans, raisins, apricots, legumes, pumpkin seeds, quinoa, broccoli, tofu, and whole grains. • Consuming 10-15 overnight soaked black raisins – HB, relieves constipation. • Along with iron rich diet add lemons, oranges, tomatoes vitamin C which helps in best absorption of iron. • Wheat + Satu flour phulka, • Sprouts (with less water), usual, sesame-karal, garlic chutney. • Masoor kulthi – Daal, soup • Carrot – cabbage- onion – kachumber, fresh buttermilk, • If want to eat rice take make by roasting. • Haldi pickle, garlic, ginger pickle • Morning- neem juice, karela, amla juice • Steam vegetables – roti- buttermilk • Tambul, supari, long, after meal . • For burning feet- cucumber with honey.	
Obesity – sthaulya – Consume low fat and low calorie food. Warm water is beneficial for drinking. • Protein diet will help to stay longer without food . so one can add cereals with high protein. • Small meals help to restore energy for a long. • Use low calorie low fat milk products . even buttermilk can be made by using more water.	

• Use salads, nimbu, amla, carrot, beet, ginger, saindhav, dhania, moong, jaggery (instead of white sugsr), pomegranate, cucumber, barly laja, cumin. • Avoid sweet fruits instead use bitter fruits like jamun, kapith. • Use roasted cereals. • Use spices adequately.	

Chapter 11

Some new concepts of food

A. Colour and food

Colours have impact on mind and body. a colourful dish stimulates one's hunger and stimulates digestive juices. Food marketing company's use such strategies which attracts the customers to buy that product.

Colour effect is seen on dosha as well as nervous system. we use specific colour therapy in specific diseases.

As red is irritating to pitta dosha, black irritates almost all three dosha. We can use this concept for specific conditions.

Artificial colours are not indicated in ayurved we can use natural food items to give colour.

Turmeric, chili's, tomato purée, coriander, pudina, leafy vegetables can be used for same purpose.

1. Yellow colour- it stimulates hunger so can be used in anorexia Indigestion or as an appetizer. Yellow food is good source of vitamin A.

Sources – Yellow Capsicum, Orange, Papaya, Banana, Mangoes,

2. Red colour – red food stimulates hunger and digestive juices. Red colour is used as a colour of attraction.
   Sources – tomatoes, radish, beet, watermelon, cherries,

3. Green colour – green is related with nature; it is fresh and cool so many of food company use these colours for natural feelings. Green colour is good for immunity, improve digestion.
   Sources – cucumber, spinach, Methi, coriander, green grapes

4. White – white colour is cooling smoothening, refreshing.
   Sources – potatoes, mushrooms, onion, radish

5. Orange – orange colour is refreshing and catchy. It is beneficial to maintain skin health, immune system.
   Sources – oranges, papaya, mangoes, pumpkin, carrots,

6. Blue – blue colour is favourite among all. Blue is important for memory and promotes healthy aging. Blue colour is used for supressing hunger to maintain weight.
   Sources – blueberries, eggplant, raisins, blue corn, blue potatoes

7. Purple – purple colour is full of antioxidants
   Sources – blueberries, cabbage, purple carrots, purple pepper
   One can have rainbow diet by planning one day one colour.

Day	Color
One -	White
Two	Red
Three	Green
Four	Orange
Five	Purple
Six	Yellow
Seven	Rainbow colour

B.   How to change food –

If a person changes a state or city he might be confused how to adapt a specific culture.

Simple rule is that when we shift in different food culture area. Don't replace new food immediately as it may cause disturbances in digestion. First two months eat according to your previous food culture then add one meal with new culture. if you can digest it easily start half new meal and half old meal. In next third month you can continue with full new food culture.

Averagely you can adapt a new food culture in 5-6 months of time period.

www.ingramcontent.com/pod-product-compliance
Lightning Source LLC
Chambersburg PA
CBHW020535290526
45786CB00002B/889